LOW BACK PAIN & SCIATICA

LOW BACK PAIN

&

SCIATICA

A PERSONALISED TREATMENT APPROACH

PAUL BOXCER

Spinal Health Publishing

British Library Cataloguing in Publication Data
A catalogue record for this book is available from the British Library.

ISBN 978-0-9562931-0-7

Typeset by Amolibros, Milverton, Somerset
This book production has been managed by Amolibros
Printed and bound by Wai Man Book Binding (China) Ltd.

About the Author

Firstly, a little information about myself. My name is Paul Boxcer and after leaving school at the age of sixteen I spent four and a half years working for a bank in the City of London. I then decided to up sticks and spend some time travelling the world. After two years of travelling around Israel, Egypt, Europe, Australia and China, I decided it was time to settle down and get some kind of career behind me. I had two goals I wanted to achieve with this new career:

1) I wanted to help people.

2) I wanted to enjoy it.

Admittedly, there was no 'eureka' moment as such but I was led into further education (back to college to get some 'A' Levels which I hadn't hung around to take the first time!) in order to pursue my new career. Fortunately, all went well and I progressed to the University of East London to complete my degree in Physiotherapy.

After attaining a BSc (Hons) degree in Physiotherapy, I worked as a physiotherapist within the NHS. Several years working around the UK were soon followed by another attack of the travel bug and I decided to spend the next two years working in Christchurch, New Zealand. During this time, I was fortunate enough to work in one of the leading sports clinics in the country. However, after two years in New Zealand the urge to come home was too strong and since then I have been working back in 'Blighty'.

During my time working as a physiotherapist, it has always intrigued me as to why some people suffering with pain get better and others do not...even though their diagnoses and subsequent treatments may be the same. This is particularly evident with individuals who suffer from low back pain and sciatica. It has been my own self-analysis of this that has culminated in me writing this book.

Contents

Introduction   *1*

The Principles of this Book   *13*

Here I explain the general structure of my book as well as
any terminology I use throughout. Some phrases within this
book are ones I tend to use from day to day and are more
likely to be specific to me as opposed to standard medical
terms.

Step One: *Red Flags*   *21*

The first and most important step to take with regard to
resolving your pain is to make sure it is musculo-skeletal in
nature, i.e. being caused by problems with muscles, joints &
soft tissue. There are also other causes of low back pain and
sciatica, and this chapter will highlight any specific signs and
symptoms that may indicate you are suffering from one of
them. If you do have any of these signs and symptoms, the
chances are there is nothing to worry about. However, it is
always best to err on the side of caution and seek professional
medical advice.

Learning Zone: *Your Lower Back and Sciatic Nerve*   *27*

This is where I explain the functional anatomy of your lower
back and sciatic nerve. I go into detail, but not too much, to

provide you with a good understanding of what the lower back looks like, as well as explanations of the bones, joints, ligaments and muscles of which it consists. I also give a description of the sciatic nerve, from where it begins and to where it travels.

Learning Zone: *Why You are Feeling Pain* 51

Any incorrect postures or movements, along with muscle imbalance, can lead to low back pain and/or sciatica. During this chapter I explain why this is so and also describe the two types of pain you are likely to be suffering from, i.e. Acute Inflammatory Pain and Mechanical Pain.

Learning Zone: *Your Own Body is the Greatest Healer* 65

Your body has an innate desire to heal itself. If you provide it with the correct conditions ***it will heal itself*** and resolve your pain. This chapter helps you understand why.

Step Two: *How to STOP Acutely Inflamed Pain* 71

If you are suffering with an acute inflammatory attack of pain, the pain will be constant and unremitting. This type of pain can result in almost intolerable surges of pain with what appears to be the simplest of movements. It will also feel as if you can do nothing at all to settle the pain down…but you can! This chapter provides you with the information and advice you need to ease this pain as quickly as possible. Apart from the great feeling of relief you will encounter, it will also enable you to move on to exercises that will completely resolve your pain.

1) Side Lying with pillows 79
2) Prone Lying with pillows 80
3) Prone Lying 80
4) Crook Lying 80
5) Lying with your feet supported on a chair 80

Step Three: *How to Optimise Your Body's Healing Potential* *85*

It is important you harness as much of your body's innate desire to heal itself as is possible, if you are to resolve your pain. In this chapter, not only do I show you how best to detect and eliminate the things that are interfering with your body's healing process, I also teach you how to detect and encourage the things that will facilitate that same healing process. This optimisation of your body's healing potential will speed up your recovery towards becoming free of pain.

Step Four: *How to Diagnose Your Pain* *99*

The crucial factor in resolving your pain is finding the correct diagnosis. This section of the book explains the functional diagnoses I use and how you can provide yourself with the correct diagnosis for your low back pain and/or sciatica. There is a reason for me putting this diagnostic stage a little later in the book. This is because prior to this, the primary goal is directed towards acutely inflamed pain, where pretty much anything and everything hurts. The main aim at that stage is simply to settle things down. As soon as the acute stage has passed, however, you will then need to diagnose your problem and become more specific with regard to the exercises you need to perform. This chapter addresses those issues.

Practical Advice: *The Influence of Regular Day-to-day*   125
Activities on Your Pain

This chapter highlights the day-to-day activities that most of us perform and how they may be preventing your body from curing itself of your pain. It also guides you to the specific section of the book that reveals the remedy to any problems you may recognise.

Practical Advice: *How Recognising Daily Patterns of Pain*   149
Will Help Cure Your Pain

Have you noticed a specific pattern that your pain tends to take, day in, day out? Maybe your pain is always better or worse first thing in the morning, or getting to sleep is always difficult. There are several typical patterns that low back pain and sciatica tend to take. All of these are covered in this chapter. If you recognise any of them, it will help you shed light on why you are encountering them and also help you to deduce from this pattern the best way to speed up your healing process.

Practical Advice: *Do Not Replace Your Bed*   159

If you are a low back pain or sciatica sufferer and finding it difficult to get a good night's sleep or waking with pain and stiffness in the morning, do not fall into the trap of replacing your bed. More often than not it is something else that is the problem and therefore replacing your bed would be an unnecessary expense. Make sure you read this chapter and look to address the cause of this problem before buying a new bed.

Learning Zone: *The Principles of Exercise*   *169*

> Before prescribing yourself with a specific exercise programme for your given diagnosis, this chapter highlights the best way to go about the exercises. For example, how many to perform, when to increase or decrease the intensity of the exercises and how, once you have cured yourself of pain, to keep yourself free from low back pain and sciatica forever.

Step Five: *Getting Moving Again*   *185*

> As your pain will have now moved away from the acute inflammatory stage, it is now time to begin exercises that will continue your improvement. These include specific exercises for your given diagnosis as well as stretching and movement exercises that will address the underlying cause of why you were suffering pain in the first place.

Treating Flexion Dominated Pain (FDP)   189
Extension Exercises for FDP:-

1) Prone Lying with Pillows   189
2) Prone Lying   190
3) Prone Lying on your Forearms/in Extension   190

Treating Extension Dominated Pain (EDP)   193
Flexion Exercises for EDP:-

1) Posterior Pelvic Tilt (Lying and Standing)   193
2) Knees to Chest   195
3) Four Point Kneeling Flexion   196
4) Forward Flexion (Sitting)   197
5) Forward Flexion (Standing)   198

Stretching & Moving Exercises: 200

1) Knee Rolls   200
2) Thoracic Rotations   201
3) Side Stretch   202

Learning Zone: *Why Muscles are the Key Factor in Eliminating Your Pain*   *205*

> Without doubt, muscles, be they either tight or weak, are the main contributor towards musculo-skeletal low back pain and sciatica. Here I will explain why.

Step Six: *Move Forward with Stretching Exercises*   *217*

> Suppleness is critical to allow your lower back and sciatic nerve to carry out your daily activities, without causing you any pain. This chapter will provide you with an array of stretching exercises, which you will be able to self prescribe for your given diagnosis, to create suppleness for any tightness you may have. This will reduce any inappropriate stresses and therefore further encourage your body's healing process.

1) Gluteal Stretch   220
2) Piriformis Stretch   221
3) Hamstring Stretch   225
4) Quadriceps Stretch   228
5) Iliopsoas Stretch   231
6) Latissimus Dorsi Stretch   232
7) Adductor Stretch   234
8) Gastrocnemius Stretch   235
9) Soleus Stretch   235

Core Stability is a phrase commonly used, which addresses the important stabilising muscles of your lower back and pelvic region. This chapter provides you with exercises that address these important muscles, thereby helping you to maintain a good posture and also have good core stability for your daily routine. These exercises also help reduce any inappropriate stresses present, further optimising your body's healing properties.

The 'Neutral Spine' Position   241
Abdominal Biased Exercises   242

1) Leg Slides with Full Support   243
2) Leg Slides without Touching the Floor   243
3) Single Knee Raise   244
4) Double Knee Raise   244
5) Leg Slides with No Support   245

Multifidus Biased Exercises   246

1) Prone Arm Raise   247
2) Prone Leg Raise   247
3) Prone 'Cross-Overs'   248
4) Four Point Kneeling Arm Raise   248
5) Four Point Kneeling Leg Raise   249
6) Four Point Kneeling 'Cross-Overs'   249

'Global' Core Stability Exercises   250

1) Bridging   251
2) Single Leg Bridging   251

I have placed this as a separate chapter and not a step as such, as these are exercise that I do not tend to prescribe a great deal. Nevertheless, I do sometimes and therefore do not wish to leave them out. The previous chapter, **Step Seven: *Move Forward with Core Stability Exercises***, is without doubt pivotal with regard to resolving your low back pain and/or sciatica, as the core stability muscles play a crucial role in the functioning of your lower back and pelvis. However, there are also other muscles that may be contributing to your pain. This chapter shows you how to strengthen these muscles, which in turn will continue to reduce any inappropriate stress across your lower back and sciatic nerve, therefore further encouraging healing to take place.

Gluteal Exercises   257

1) Bridging   257
2) Single Leg Bridging   257
3) Bridging on a Chair   258
4) Small Knee Bends   259
5) Lunges   260
6) Step Ups   261

Hamstring Exercises   262

1) Bridging   262
2) Single Leg Bridging   262
3) Bridging on a Chair   263
4) Lunges   265
5) Step Ups   266

Quadriceps Exercises   267

1) Small Knee Bends   267
2) Lunges   268
3) Step-Ups   269

And Finally…

Old Wives' Tales   *271*

> If you are fed up with everyone you know having an opinion on how to ease your pain, it is imperative you read this chapter. I will highlight these old wives' tales and give you my opinion as to whether any of them have any validity.

Conclusion   *295*

Appendix I: *Glossary of Diagnostic Terms*   *299*

> Many people are given a diagnosis from a health professional that may as well be written in a foreign language. This appendix will explain in lay terms what these diagnostic terms mean.

Appendix II: *Glossary of Terms*   *313*

> This appendix is a glossary of any medical terms used throughout the book.

A massive hearfelt thank-you to my parents, who have been so supportive to me over the years. I have no doubt I would not be the person I am today without that support.

Foreword by Gail Forrester-Gale

For ease of reference throughout this foreword, when referring to Low back pain (LBP), it will also be with regards to sciatica (pain felt in the leg) as well.

Low back pain (LBP), with or without leg pain (sciatica), is an extremely common disorder affecting around one third of the UK adult population each year. Anyone who has experienced an episode of LBP for any length of time will appreciate the distressing, disabling and frustrating nature of the condition. On the whole, the majority of LBP is self limiting, although it is traditionally managed in the western world by health care professionals using a range of manual or other therapeutic techniques. These commonly employed treatment approaches have variable success rates and so despite the intense research activity that has been devoted to the management of LBP over the last twenty or thirty years there is still a lack of consensus regarding the best forms of treatment for this disorder. What is well accepted, however, is that people with LBP who have poor physical function, who are afraid of moving their back, who are anxious, in distress or who have negative feelings about their LBP are more disabled by their pain and more likely to have a poor outcome. Conversely, people who have a good understanding of their LBP and who feel empowered to adopt an active approach in its management frequently do well. Therefore, it is generally agreed that education, information, advice and safe levels of appropriate activity play an important role in the successful management and resolution of LBP and sciatica.

Of all the people that suffer from LBP annually in the UK only about one in five will consult their GP, which means that a large number of people are trying to manage their back pain independently. This can be a bewildering task especially given the abundance of information available and the array of alternative practitioners on hand to treat the disorder. It is no wonder then that individuals with LBP often find it perplexing and difficult to know what to do for the best and where to turn for sensible, appropriate and effective advice.

This is where this book comes in. *Low Back Pain and Sciatica – A Personalised Treatment Approach* has been written by a physiotherapist with many years of experience in the musculoskeletal field who has devoted much time listening to and observing patients with LBP. His initial curiosity was triggered by the fact that some patients with LBP recovered whilst others with seemingly similar LBP took longer to improve or did not recover at all, despite them receiving similar types of treatment. This lead him to believe it was not necessarily what he did as a health care practitioner that made the difference but what the individual with LBP did or didn't do themselves and how their lifestyle and daily activities contributed to their disorder that mattered. Based on these observations, the author firmly believes that given the right conditions the body has an innate ability and desire to heal itself. Consequently, the biggest impact on the resolution of LBP is what individuals do themselves in order to provide their body with the optimal conditions for healing to occur.

This fundamental belief forms the basis from which the approach adopted throughout the book has evolved. The author strongly emphasises the key role individuals have to play in the resolution of their LBP, placing importance on them being in control and learning how to manage and relieve their own pain. This is achieved in the book through an easy-to-follow, step by step approach in which relevant knowledge, appropriate tools and simple guidance are logically presented in order to provide individuals with a good understanding of their LBP and sensible strategies to facilitate self-healing and pain resolution.

Low Back Pain and Sciatica – A Personalised Treatment Approach is a thorough and systematic book that is divided into helpful sections to enable the individual to identify conditions that will impact on and promote the body's natural healing process. The first few sections are devoted to self-diagnosis and are designed to help individuals identify the general cause of their LBP and to rule out any serious underlying conditions that may be causing their

LBP and therefore may require a medical consultation. Subsequent sections aim to develop the individual's understanding of LBP and to allow the individual logically to match the most appropriate form of management to the type of LBP they are suffering from. From these sections you will learn what you can do to alleviate your pain, how you can safely increase your activity levels, what daily activities may be contributing to your LBP and what simple lifestyle changes you can make in order to provide the optimal environment for healing to occur. Additional sections challenge the common myths that surround LBP, address frequently asked questions about LBP and outline general exercise programmes that are safe and appropriate for LBP sufferers.

This book was written primarily to help individuals suffering from LBP and sciatica. It was therefore the author's intention to provide a 'patient friendly' book which was largely free of medical jargon and did not continually refer to the current evidence. It is, however, appropriate to note at this point that all the advice and guidance provided within this book is in line with the current national guidelines for the management of LBP as reported by the National Institute for Health and Clinical Excellence (2009). These national guidelines are the result of lengthy and careful consideration of all the current available research evidence on LBP and its management by the country's leading experts and provide the framework for the management of LBP by the NHS. Consequently, the approach adopted in this book reflects the best of current clinical practice and research evidence.

In summary, this book provides a logical, straightforward and accessible guide to the self-management and resolution of LBP and sciatica. It is refreshing in its simplicity with up-to-date, evidence-based advice and guidance presented in a format that is easy to follow and apply. The author should be commended on the provision of such a helpful text for sufferers of LBP.

Gail Forrester-Gale

Introduction

Thank you for taking the time to read this book. You will not regret it as it offers you a no-nonsense, commonsense approach to resolving your low back pain and/or sciatica, with minimal disruption to your lifestyle. No trendy exercises, gym programmes or special dietary needs: just a simple 'back to basics' approach in which you leave all the hard work to the greatest healer of all – your own body.

Yes, that's right. Your body is equipped with the most fantastic and efficient healing qualities known to man; the problem is we do not always provide it with the correct conditions it needs to work to the best of its ability.

The human body has an innate desire to heal itself. Whether you have fallen over and cut yourself, broken a bone or even suffered some kind of serious illness, the body will always strive to heal itself...when we develop low back pain or sciatica, it is no different.

By reading this book, you will begin to learn all the things to do (and not to do) for your body to begin healing itself. Consequently, as your body heals itself it will become stronger, resulting in your pain diminishing and the chances of you suffering further episodes of pain decreasing.

My aim in writing this book is to provide a succinct explanation of how and why we tend to develop low back pain and sciatica. More importantly, you will also be given the knowledge to self diagnose your specific problem. From this you will progress to prescribing yourself with an appropriate exercise programme, tailored to your specific problem, in order to alleviate your pain completely.

During my research, I found many books which provided plenty of statistics and general information on low back pain and sciatica. For example, how many working days are lost due to low back pain, the amount of money it costs the economy, information about the numerous things which could go wrong with the back and also lists of exercises which could be performed... but that was as good as it got.

Just a simple list of statistics, potential problems and exercises, all of which can be found on the internet these days anyway. I found no guidance as to which exercises will help *your* specific problem and probably, equally importantly, those exercises which may aggravate *your pain* and therefore make it worse.

A classic example of this arose when I was reading one book, which suggested if your pain is particularly bad first thing in the morning you should avoid sitting for the first couple of hours. Although I can see the thinking behind this, I'm afraid I cannot agree at all with the underlying logic. Okay, so by not sitting for the first couple of hours you may well find your pain does ease a little, BUT you may also find it gets worse!

In a nutshell, such information is simply providing a solution that would be applicable for certain types of pain but not for others.

Continuing from this example, it is equally important to establish why you are waking in pain in the first place. Ultimately, we need to address the *cause of the problem* and not just the signs and symptoms.

That's where this book truly comes into its own. Not only can I assure you it will constantly be looking to find the cause of your pain, it will also be encouraging you to ask yourself specific, tailored questions. The answers to these questions will be *unique to you* and they will therefore *give you the knowledge* to provide yourself with a functional diagnosis and subsequent exercises for your pain. You will therefore gain the specific knowledge of your own back to be able to maintain and take care of it for the rest of your life.

In essence, I have written this book with the intention of it being a transcript of how my assessment and subsequent treatment would go if you were with me in the physiotherapy department, all in front of you in print so you can dip in and out of it as needed.

So why did I write this book?

During my time as a physiotherapist, I have always paid particular attention to how individuals with low back pain and/or sciatica respond to their treatment.

The more I have observed, the further I have moved away from the traditional approach of using electrotherapy, mobilising and manipulating the spine to a more 'holistic' approach where the patient's lifestyle and what they generally do and do not do is taken into account.

This all started when I became intrigued as to why some people, who presented with similar problems and were given similar treatments, would respond differently to the treatment I had provided them with, i.e. some would make a 100 per cent recovery and others would not. This made me analyse everything in more detail:

i)   Were the diagnoses correct and similar?
ii) Were the treatments exactly the same?
iii) Were the patients carrying out the exercises as requested and following the advice I had given?

As I did this, and noted the results, it was quite evident it was not what I was doing that was the key, but rather what the patient was doing outside of physiotherapy that was the critical factor.

> *It is important to mention that I saw this as a fault on my part and not the patient's, as it was I who had failed to pick up on these things and therefore educate the patient accordingly.*

As a result of this, I began to place more emphasis on listening carefully to each patient, enabling myself to understand better their lifestyle and daily activities. This is crucial because, after all, it is likely to be their lifestyle and daily activities that have contributed to their pain in the first place.

By doing this, it allowed me to elicit any particular aggravating factors which may be hindering the patient's healing process, as well as discovering any easing factors that would facilitate it.

Before I knew it, more and more of my time was spent listening to each patient. This was followed by us working together to determine the next steps to take and appropriate advice to give in order to eradicate their pain as soon as possible.

In short, I was taking more of a 'hands off' approach to my treatment. The irony of it was, the less hands-on treatment I was carrying out, the more time I actually spent with the patient in the treatment cubicle. This was because the process itself was often detective-like in its nature, as I tried to unravel the things which were both causing the individual their pain and also preventing it from getting better.

However, although I seemed to be spending more time during each individual treatment session, the results being obtained were much better. I needed to see each patient less frequently and equally, if not more importantly, the patients were now managing their own pain as opposed to relying on me to 'get their pain better'. That's not to say I didn't perform any hands-on treatment at all, as there were obviously occasions that dictated a need to treat someone's back manually; it was just that these occasions seemed to become less frequent.

I also started to see results just by giving people the appropriate advice over the phone. If a patient came in to see me and I was confident there needed to be no hands-on treatment, I would often give them instructions as to how I intended to conduct their exercises, along with being as specific as I could with regard to any potential problems they may encounter. I would then offer to call them within a week or two to see how they were progressing.

When I called them I would ask how they were, at what stage they were at with their exercises and if they had any particular problems. Depending upon how they were doing, I would then guide them as to how to progress.

More often than not this would be enough for the patient to have the confidence and knowledge to treat their own pain. Consequently, they would continue to manage it until they had recovered and therefore would not need to visit the physiotherapy department again.

That isn't to say this approach worked perfectly every time. Sometimes a patient would reach a plateau that could not be resolved with a telephone conversation. If this occurred, I would invite them in for another appointment, during which a situation would normally arise where once again no hands-on treatment was needed; just a check on the exercises and guidance in the right direction as to how to progress. The point is I was beginning to treat the majority of my patients in this way.

The difference with this book is this: rather than me having to call you and advise you on how to progress, all of the knowledge and information you need is here in writing. You can just read it as you see fit. If you do find you reach a plateau, you simply read through specific chapters again in order to see how to push things further forward and kick start the body's healing process into action again. All will be explained in due course.

An equally important bonus for this approach was that, by being more 'hands off' and concentrating more on self education, I was handing the responsibility back to the patient. By doing this, it was giving them a further understanding of how their back worked and why it was causing them pain.

Therefore, not only were they curing themselves and reducing the risk of future episodes of pain, but in the unlikely event they did suffer another episode, they would know exactly what to do in order to resolve it as soon as possible. In short, the individuals concerned were now able to manage their own body for the rest of their lives, rather than relying on other health professionals to 'fix' their back for them.

This addresses one of the major frustrations I encounter when treating individuals with low back pain and/or sciatica. With my unique approach, more often than not the problem can be resolved with appropriate advice and exercises. If this is the case, the individual concerned will follow their plan accordingly and completely resolve their pain.

However, in the unlikely event their pain returns, they will have the knowledge and know-how to think about why they are suffering with pain and therefore take appropriate action. This will likely involve temporarily modifying certain activities, as well as providing themselves with any exercises they need to perform. If this action is taken straight away, it will not be long before the pain disappears.

The alternative to this is the individual who seeks manual therapy for his or her problem. Should this treatment approach work but they are given no advice on how to look after their back or exercises to perform, what are they going to think if their pain returns? I can almost guarantee you it will be something along the lines of "Oh, I need to see Mr/Mrs X again to have my back 'fixed'" or words to that effect.

If the causative factors (usually incorrect posture along with tight and/

or weak muscles) are resulting in the joints of the lower back stiffening up then yes, a manipulation here and there may loosen those joints a little and make you feel better. However, the underlying problem as to why these joints stiffened will still exist and over time will cause your back to tighten up and become painful again. The individual will then think he or she needs another trip to their practitioner to 're-align' their back.

The irony of this is that if these individuals have not been given the appropriate advice and exercises, **which are all covered within this book**, the chances of them having had the cause of their problem addressed is unlikely and therefore the chances of them developing pain again is quite high.

This will set up a vicious cycle, where they seek someone to 'fix' their back every time they begin to feel pain, instead of addressing the cause of the problem and eliminating it completely. As a result of the cause not being addressed, it is likely their low back will become stiffer and/or weaker, which will increase the chances of further episodes of pain occurring, resulting in more trips back to the practitioner in order to have their back 'fixed' again. I am sure you can see how this vicious cycle continues from here…

This is a problem you will not encounter with this book. Addressing the cause of your pain is imperative and also surprisingly straightforward, as long as you know what to look for.

Finding the cause of your pain and knowing how to address it is exactly what you will learn to do by reading this book.

So isn't seeing someone for my pain good enough?

It should be good enough providing you are treated appropriately. Unfortunately, I do not believe this is always the case. However, even if it is good enough, I believe that many people are 'over treated' where manual hands-on treatment is continued, when a simple exercise programme would suffice.

My belief is that any individual seeking treatment for their low back pain or sciatica will be seen by their therapist three times per week as an *absolute maximum*. Let's say each session is for 30 minutes, although the actual hands-on treatment would be significantly less than this; multiply that by 3 and you have 1½ hours of treatment per week.

If we multiply the 24 hours in a day by the 7 days in a week, we are given a figure of 168 hours. Therefore, this individual would have their back 'treated' for only 1½ hours from a total of 168 hours throughout the week. In percentage terms this equates to less than 0.9 per cent of 'treatment'.

To have your back 'treated' a maximum of 0.9 per cent of the time is not sufficient if you wish to optimise the rate at which it can heal itself, and, of equal importance, if you wish to decrease the risk of enduring further episodes of back pain.

> *It is important I highlight that this figure of 168 hours is relevant, even though up to a third of this time may be spent sleeping. If you are sleeping in a position which is comfortable for you, as opposed to one which aggravates your pain, your body will heal itself sooner. It is important to remember that…*
>
> **Night Time is Prime Healing Time!**

By me adopting this more thorough, holistic approach, I've had patients who have been able to return to sport, gym and general exercise after years of believing they would never be able to, simply because they had now developed confidence in their own back.

Of equal, if not greater, satisfaction was one particular patient who returned to work following years of living on disability benefit after being labelled 'disabled' because of his low back pain.

Did this particular patient become pain-free? In actual fact he did not, although his pain did reduce dramatically. What happened was that he gained the confidence and trust in knowing how to look after and listen to his own body. He therefore had the confidence to go out and gain employment in an appropriate line of work, instead of being too frightened because of being told many years before by a consultant that 'if he wasn't careful he would end up in a wheelchair' – an outrageous and untrue statement to make!

I have mentioned this particular patient, even though he did not make a 100 per cent recovery from his low back pain, because by adopting what I consider to be the simple strategies given throughout this book, the impact on this individual's quality of life and self esteem were immense.

This example was particularly satisfying, as when we first met he was sceptical as to whether physiotherapy would provide him with any benefit. This was because he had been treated many times before over the years and had had very little success. However, previous treatments had given him no education on how to listen to, look after and manage his own back.

This patient actually confided in me afterwards that the only reason he attended physiotherapy was because his General Practitioner (GP) had been quite insistent on it and he was concerned he may lose his benefits! The irony being that he no longer needed benefits afterwards as he returned to work.

Take action as soon as possible!

Any health professional will tell you that one of the biggest obstacles encountered when treating low back pain or sciatica is the longer the pain has been around, the more difficult it is to resolve (although that's not saying it's impossible, it just makes it a little bit harder).

I often see patients within the physiotherapy department where the individual concerned has been through the process of seeing their GP and being prescribed anti-inflammatories. They then return to their GP several times afterwards with no improvement and yet they are prescribed more pain killers and/or anti-inflammatories.

Eventually, because there is no improvement, they are sent for an unnecessary x-ray which comes back negative, although diagnoses such as Degenerative Disc Disease, Spondylosis, Wear and Tear, etc. may be used (see **Appendix I:** *Glossary of Diagnostic Terms*). Following this, they are then sent to see a consultant, who has nothing to offer and finally they are referred to physiotherapy!

The timescale for all this can be as much as a year or more, plenty of time for any tight muscles to become even tighter and any weak ones to become even weaker. Little wonder then that this type of pain is more difficult to treat than the person who attends the physiotherapy department much sooner.

I am hoping that by writing this book and giving you a step-by-step approach on how to diagnose and treat your own pain, you will gain the confidence to take action immediately and therefore avoid being caught up in this unnecessary cycle. This will not only resolve any current problems you may have, but also empower you with the knowledge and ability to take immediate action if you do happen to develop any kind of pain in the future.

> *If you read this book and take action, I am confident you will not even need to make an appointment to see your GP!*

I also hope to break down the medical language barriers that patients may encounter. For example:

> ➤ **The 40 year old being told he has the 'spine of an 80 year old'.**

> ➤ **Someone in their 50s being stopped in their tracks because they have 'Spondylosis' of the spine (basically wear and tear which we all begin to develop as we pass through our late 20s and 30s).**

> ➤ **The outrageous claims that individuals have to 'stop work/change their lifestyle' otherwise they will end up in a wheelchair!**

These are quotes I have heard numerous times from patients who have been referred to me after seeing their GP or Orthopaedic Consultant.

Without a shadow of a doubt, the majority of low back pain and sciatica from which the general population suffer is down to a few repeated, incorrect postures or movements being placed upon the spine, along with a muscle imbalance involving either tight and/or weak muscles.

These combine to place increased stresses upon the lower back and nerves, which ultimately lead to the body's pain threshold levels being breached and therefore the feeling of pain. Following this a vicious cycle often results, whereby incorrect movements and postures encourage tight and weak muscles and the tight and weak muscles encourage incorrect movements and postures.

If these problems are addressed – *and this book will show you how to do so* – there is no reason why your pain should not resolve itself thanks to the human body's wonderful healing process...

I truly believe this book can cure you of the pain you are currently suffering.

Therefore I shall keep you no longer and let you read on.

Enjoy the rest of this book and, more importantly, a pain-free future.

Paul

The Principles of this Book

Before you begin reading this book, I would just like to outline the structure upon which I have written it and also highlight some of the terminology I use from time to time.

First, the structure upon which this book is written: I have tried to make it simple, step by step, and not too complicated. One step leads to another as you are guided seamlessly through the book and back to a life free of pain: I have produced **7 Steps** to enable you to do this.

However, in order to understand fully and make the most of these steps, I have also included some chapters where I explain things in a little more detail. I have placed these within chapters entitled **Learning Zone** as that is what each will do; that is, teach and give you more of an understanding either with regard to the anatomy of the lower back and sciatic nerve itself or with regard to how I expect you to use this book to optimise your body's healing.

Therefore, in summary, the **7 Steps** given to freeing yourself from your pain are chapters in which you are encouraged to do something. For example, checking your signs and symptoms to make sure it is musculo-skeletal pain you are suffering with is explained in **Step One:** *Red Flags*. You are shown how to diagnose your pain during **Step Four:** *How to Diagnose Your Pain* and you will also learn how to prescribe yourself with specific stretching exercises in **Step Six:** *Move Forward with Stretching Exercises*.

To complement this, there are **Learning Zone** chapters that are more concerned with you gaining an understanding of your lower back and/or sciatic nerve. For example, *Your Lower Back and Sciatic Nerve* describes the functional anatomy of this part of the body; *Your Own Body is the Greatest Healer* explains why your body has an innate desire to heal itself and *Why Muscles are the Key Factor in Eliminating Your Pain* explains why muscles, be they tight or weak, play such a fundamental role in the cause of low back pain and sciatica.

I also have three chapters under the title **Practical Advice:** these chapters will provide you with vital information on how you can benefit from looking at and analysing your typical day-to-day activities and postures.

Finally I have two chapters at the end of this book which are a kind of aside to the rest of the book, but may play an important part in resolving your pain. Those two chapters are ***Specific Strengthening Outside of Core Stability*** and ***Old Wives' Tales.***

The former of these two chapters gives you some simple strengthening exercises for the larger muscles, such as the Gluteals, Hamstrings and Quadriceps, where weakness may be influencing your low back pain or sciatica. I do not tend to prescribe these exercises very often, but nevertheless I do sometimes and therefore did not want to leave them out of this book.

The last chapter ***Old Wives' Tales*** is a chapter where I share with you my opinion on advice you may have been given by friends and family. I am often asked about these in the physiotherapy department, as such advice can be confusing or misleading. Therefore I have given my opinion on these within this chapter.

With regard to the terminology used throughout this book, I have done my utmost to eliminate medical jargon. However, I have tended to adopt a few little phrases myself over the years of being a physiotherapist. I will now go on to highlight the ones I know I am guilty of in order to forewarn you.

Back Pain: I will often refer to your back pain throughout this book, which is understandable as that's probably why you have purchased it in the first place. However, when I mention back pain I do not mean just your low back pain, but also any other pain which is being referred from your lower back to other parts of your body, typically into the buttock, leg and maybe foot area.

Sciatica: This is any pain which passes down through the buttock and/or down the back of the leg which is emanating from the Sciatic Nerve. It is important to note that sciatica is not a diagnostic term, only a descriptive one. Two individuals may be suffering with pain down the back of the leg, i.e. sciatica, but there may be two completely different reasons as to why they are suffering with this pain. Consequently, it will mean the treatment principles will also be different in each case.

Pain and Stretching: I will often use the words *pain* and *stretching*. When you carry out any kind of movement or exercise, or if you are in any kind of static posture, I will often ask what it is you can feel with regard to your back (remember, this also means your buttock, leg and foot). I will be primarily enquiring as to whether it feels *painful* or whether you feel more of a *stretching* sensation. This is because when treating low back pain or sciatica, I am always looking to divide any kind of sensation you feel into one of these two categories.

However, there are numerous sensations which can be encompassed by these two words. For example, *pain* could also be described as being one of the following sensations:

Aching, Soreness, Hurting, Throbbing, etc.

Whereas a *stretching* sensation could be described as:

Pulling, Tightness, Stiffness, Restriction, etc.

Therefore, whenever I ask you what you may be feeling, ultimately I will be looking for you to place that sensation into one of the two categories – *Pain* or *Stretching.* However, you may use different terminology to describe either of those two sensations. That's fine as long as you can distinguish between the two.

It is equally important to note that sometimes you may feel more than one sensation. For example, the overriding sensation maybe one of pain, yet there may also be a feeling of stretching with it. Under these circumstances I would say the given movement/activity is a painful one and therefore be guided by that with regard to how you continue.

Alternatively, you may feel a strong stretching sensation, yet as you stretch or move further it starts to become painful. This time I would say that stretching is the overriding factor and once again be guided by this with regard to how you continue.

Ultimately, be guided by your signs and symptoms, i.e. what your body is telling you. You will realise as you read this book that your body will always strive to tell you what it does and does not like. If you listen to how it is responding to certain activities/exercises, you will not go far wrong.

The human body is unique, it is not a machine

You will also see I often use phrases such as 'rule of thumb', 'tend to', 'listen to your body' and 'gut instinct'. Although it may seem as if I am sitting on the fence, since I'm not giving specific instructions on what to do, nothing could be further from the truth. It is quite simply because the human body is not a machine.

Although the medical/health profession try to make the study of the human body a science (and I fully understand why), the human body is not a machine. It is for this reason I believe it is not and never will be a true science. I have personally found this to be what I consider a fault of many people who work within the health profession. I have encountered many colleagues who try to have their patients' condition fit with what a text book says... and if it doesn't? Well, that's down to the patient; they are either making things up or aren't explaining things well enough!

Whenever a patient sees me in the physiotherapy department, without exception I believe whatever they tell me is 100 per cent true. How do I know? Because they are the only ones who know and can feel what they are feeling. Who am I to judge and believe what they are saying is not true, when I have absolutely no way of knowing what they are feeling? The fact is, no matter how much theoretical knowledge we may have, there is still a huge amount to learn about the human body and no one else can understand and feel what they are feeling as well as a particular individual does.

> *Being part of the health profession, I can confidently say we now know a fantastic amount about the human body. Truth be told though, the fantastic amount we do understand is probably tiny when compared to what we have yet to learn.*

I may have laboured the point a little here, but what I am trying to say is that it is impossible to say to you, whether it is by reading this book or if you were in the physiotherapy department standing beside me, "Perform such and such exercise and your back will feel better." You always need to be guided by how your body responds to those exercises, and I stress this in my book.

It is also one of the reasons why this is not a book full of references to research. Firstly, it is because I want it to be as free from medical jargon as possible. If I were to make references towards certain research, you can rest assured the research itself would be full of medical terminology. However, the other reason is that the results from any given research may not be appropriate for your specific problem. Remember, the body is not a machine and we are all built differently.

Research is all based upon the laws of probability, therefore there is a possible chance (even though it may not be seen as statistically significant) that any given piece of research will not be applicable to you. My belief therefore is to *listen to your body.* If you are performing a particular activity or exercise and your pain is improving, your body is obviously beginning to heal itself, therefore continue with whatever it is you are doing. If, on the other hand, your pain increases, your body obviously does not like what you are doing and the healing process is being interfered with. Consequently you would need to ease off or stop performing that particular activity or exercise.

If research suggests you should perform a certain exercise or sit in a certain way in order to resolve your pain, yet when you do this your pain gets worse, does it make sense to continue to do so simply because the research says you should? Of course it doesn't.

I do not want you to think I am being dismissive of research. Without doubt it plays a vital role in helping us to understand more about the human body. I am just trying to say that ultimately you need to listen to how your body responds to any exercises you perform or activities you carry out. As I mentioned above, if your body likes what you are doing, your pain will subside and the injured structures will begin to heal themselves and become stronger. If, however, it does not like what you are doing, your pain will increase and those same structures will stay sensitive and painful.

It is equally important I assure you that this book can be completely supported by theory with regard to why I ask you to treat your pain the way I do. I do not want you to think everything in this book is anecdotal. All of the advice I give and the exercises I ask you to perform have sound theory behind them, all of which is explained in the relevant chapters. However, I also understand we are all unique and therefore may respond differently to the same advice and exercises. It is crucial we acknowledge this and respond accordingly.

The main 'research' as such behind this book is over thirteen years of experience and appropriate theory I have been using for treating people with low back pain and sciatica. From this, I have been able to analyse both what the patients and I have been doing and monitor what the outcomes have been. It is this analysis which has led me to the fundamental principle of this book...

If we provide the body with the correct conditions, it will heal itself.

I find this to be a very common sense approach, and I have had many patients say, *"Oh, it's common sense really,"* when I have explained these principles to them and their pain has resolved.

Finally, you will often find I repeat myself quite a bit throughout this book. Whenever you notice this, it is not due to a lack of proof reading; rather, an overriding need for me to emphasise that point. So if you keep on reading it, it must be important!

I hope everything has been explained sufficiently before you proceed. However, do not over-concern yourself if you are still a little unsure, as each chapter contains continued explanations.

We will begin with **Step One: *Red Flags*** which is an important section that ***you must read***. It covers any specific signs and symptoms you may be suffering from, which could indicate your pain is not a simple musculo-skeletal problem. After that chapter, we will then move forward with regard to curing your pain.

Step One:

Red Flags

Before I go any further, it is imperative I highlight what are referred to as **Red Flags**.

By red flags, we mean this is a warning sign that further investigations *may* be needed. The reason I have highlighted 'may' is because I do not wish to worry you into thinking something is definitely wrong. It is, however, an indication that the pain you are suffering may not be a simple musculo-skeletal one, which is what this book has been written to treat.

If you have any of the following signs or symptoms, you need to seek a health professional for a thorough assessment before proceeding further.

CAUDA EQUINA SYNDROME (CES)

At approximately the level of the first/second lumbar vertebra, the spinal cord itself finishes and the nerves form a group together referred to as the Cauda Equina, Latin for 'horse's tail', which it is said to resemble. If there is any kind of compression on the nerves in this region, typically by a prolapsed disc, it does not allow these nerves to function correctly. Typical signs and symptoms would be as follows:

Decreased Bladder and Bowel Control

The group of nerves concerned provide you with conscious control of your bladder and bowel movements. If for any reason you feel you have decreased control over your bladder or bowel, you may be suffering with CES. These symptoms may include difficulty emptying your bladder or bowel or the opposite where you find it difficult to stop yourself from emptying your bladder or bowel.

Saddle Paraesthesia (numbness and/or 'pins and needles')

These same nerves also provide you with feeling between your legs, or what we often refer to as the 'saddle' area. You may feel numbness or pins and needles in this area, i.e. in between the legs, genitalia, inner thigh or buttock area. Some people have described it as feeling 'funny' or 'different' when they wipe themselves after having been to the toilet.

Pain in the saddle area

This same saddle area where you can suffer with paraesthesia may also be a region where you suffer pain.

Sexual Dysfunction

This could be in the form of impotence or loss of ejaculation/orgasm.

If you feel you may be suffering with CES, it is important you seek ***immediate medical advice***. Contact your GP immediately and inform them of your signs and symptoms and wait for their advice as to the next step you should take. If, for whatever reason, you are unable to speak to your GP, visit your local Accident & Emergency (A&E) Department.

Severe pain and subsequent medication can also give similar signs and symptoms to CES, for example:

i)   If you are suffering with intense low back pain, it is sometimes difficult to go to the toilet, as even the slightest strain will increase your pain.

ii) Some pain-relieving medications can result in quite severe constipation, once again meaning you are unable to go to the toilet even though you may feel you want to.

Therefore, if your bladder or bowel is not functioning as it normally does, it is not necessarily because you are suffering with CES, it may be because of the pain you are in or the medication you are taking. Nevertheless, if you are in any doubt, it is important you seek professional medical advice as soon as possible, starting with your GP or visiting A&E if your GP is not available.

UNEXPLAINED WEIGHT LOSS

If you feel you have lost a significant amount of weight over the previous few weeks or months and you cannot explain why, you need to visit your GP so they can look into this in more detail. This is simply because if your eating and exercising habits have not changed a great deal, then your weight should not fluctuate too much either. If you are losing weight, there may be a reason for this, and this in turn may be responsible for your pain.

FEVER AND NIGHT SWEATS

If you feel you are suffering with a prolonged fever and/or night sweats, I suggest you visit your GP as soon as possible.

HISTORY OF CANCER

I do not wish to worry you unduly, but if you have a history of cancer and your pain is not settling down, make an appointment to see your GP. It does not necessarily mean they are related, but you should seek professional advice to make sure.

PROGRESSIVE NEUROLOGICAL DEFICIT

I strongly suggest that if you have any neurological deficit, typically pins and needles, numbness and/or weakness, you need to visit your GP as soon as possible.

Of all the signs and symptoms I have covered within this section, the feeling of pins and needles or numbness on their own are not true Red Flags. It is a complaint I hear many times each week. Any kind of irritation upon a nerve, whether it is by a prolapsed disc or quite simply a tight muscle, can lead to pins and needles and/or numbness, anywhere from your lower back down to the tips of your toes.

If a patient arrives complaining of either of these, I am not unduly concerned and treat it as a common symptom of low back pain and/or sciatica. However, I still carry out the appropriate tests. This is because although very rare, it can be indicative of other complaints and is therefore best checked out professionally.

SUMMARY

All of the Red Flags given in this chapter are rare. However, that is not a reason to be complacent. The only Red Flag I would class as a medical emergency would be *Cauda Equina Syndrome.* If you feel you may be suffering with this, it is important to speak to your GP as soon as possible. If your GP is not able to see or speak to you, visit your local A&E Department.

The chances of it being anything serious are slim. Of the thousands of patients I have seen, I have yet to encounter anyone with CES. Nevertheless, it is a potential medical emergency and therefore needs to be assessed by a health professional.

If you feel your signs and symptoms fit any of the other conditions mentioned, it is still important to speak to your GP as soon as you can, but it should not be seen as a medical emergency.

The next chapter is **Learning Zone: *Your Lower Back and Sciatic Nerve*.** Here, you will be introduced to all of the functional anatomy you need to know about with regard to your lower back and sciatic nerve. This increased knowledge will give you more of an understanding as to why you are suffering pain, which in turn will enable you to resolve it and move forward pain-free.

Learning Zone:

Your Lower Back and Sciatic Nerve

As I do with much of this book, I am going to move away from convention and provide you with what I will consistently refer to as the *functional information* required. This chapter will cover the functional anatomy of your lower back, sciatic nerve and associated muscles, joints and ligaments.

By *functional*, I mean providing all the relevant information you need to know in order to resolve your pain and go about your day-to-day activities as you did before. I personally feel that too many books go into far too much detail about the anatomy of the lower back. In addition to this, they also use far too much medical jargon. For example, I could go on to explain and provide you with detailed anatomy that shows the posterior aspect of the spine and how it contains the Supraspinous and Interspinous ligaments as well as the Ligamentum Flavum which all help to stabilise the spine, but is this necessary?

Do you need to know that much detail?

My experience tells me the typical patients I see day-in, day-out, do not. Yes, they do wish to understand the fundamental, functional anatomy of the back, how it moves and why they are suffering pain. However, if I explain and show them there are ligaments at the back of the spine that help provide it with stability, this is usually more than enough. If they wish me to explain in more detail I am happy to oblige, although to date, no one ever has. Therefore, I will explain in this chapter the key functional anatomy you need to know in order to cure yourself of your pain.

Please do not get bogged down trying to understand fully and remember all that is written within this chapter. Truth be told, you do not really need to know any of it! The way I have written this book will guide you seamlessly through how to treat and resolve your pain according to the cause and subsequent signs and symptoms of your problem. However, I have found people can relate to the advice given if they have a greater understanding of how and why their back works the way it does.

I suppose my point here is read through this chapter, enjoy it as you gain a greater knowledge and understanding of the functional anatomy of your body, but the only thing I want you to remember is that there is not a test at the end of it! As you continue to read through this book, you may find references to certain muscles or joints which you are not sure of. No problem. Just flick back to this chapter and remind yourself.

This chapter is primarily descriptive in nature, in that it explains where the structures are and their particular action/function. Although I may touch on how a certain structure can be a source/cause of pain, that is not the aim of the chapter and a more detailed explanation of potential causes of pain is given in the chapter **Learning Zone:** *Why Muscles are the Key Factor in Eliminating Your Pain*.

In **Appendix II:** *Glossary of Terms* you will find a glossary which covers any medical terms used throughout this book. However, I have covered a few here for this chapter which will save you flicking backwards and forwards.

GLOSSARY

ABDUCTION

The movement where any joint or limb (with regard to this chapter the hip or leg) is taken away from the body and out to the side. The opposite of Adduction.

ADDUCTION

The movement where any joint or limb (with regard to this chapter the hip or leg) is taken back towards the side of the body. The opposite of Abduction.

ANTERIOR

The front of your body.

ANTERIOR ROTATION

Where the top part of the pelvis moves forwards in relation to the bottom part of the pelvis: for example, if you were to lie on your back with your knees bent and tried to arch your lower back upwards away from the floor. The opposite of Posterior Rotation.

ARTICULAR SURFACE

The surface of each adjacent bone that make contact with another to form a joint.

ARTICULATE

To form a joint with, i.e. two bones articulate with each other to form a joint.

BILATERAL

Applying to both sides, i.e. left and right.

EXTENSION

With regard to the low back, this refers to the action of leaning backwards. When in relation to your hip, this is the action of taking your upper leg backwards so as to pass behind you. Extension is the opposite movement to Flexion.

EXTERNALLY ROTATES

The process of turning a limb out away from the body. With regard to the hip, imagine lying flat on your back and 'rolling' your leg outwards. The opposite of Internally Rotates.

FLEXION

With regard to the low back, this refers to the action of bending forward, as if to touch your toes. When in relation to your hip, this is the action of bringing your knee towards your chest. Flexion is the opposite movement to Extension.

INTERNALLY ROTATES

The process of turning a limb in towards the body. With regard to the hip, imagine lying flat on your back and 'rolling' your leg inwards towards your other leg. The opposite to Externally Rotates.

KYPHOSIS

The natural curve in the Thoracic Spine when viewed from the side.

LORDOSIS

The natural curve in the Lumbar and Cervical Spine when viewed from the side.

NERVE ROOTS

This is the name given to the point where some of the nerves of the spinal cord leave the vertebral column. The nerve root L1 leaves the vertebral column between the first and second lumbar vertebra, i.e. between L1 and L2. Each nerve root can join other nerve roots to form a peripheral nerve. For example, the nerve roots of L4–S3 join together to form the sciatic nerve.

POSTERIOR

The back of your body.

POSTERIOR ROTATION

Where the top part of the pelvis moves backwards in relation to the bottom part of the pelvis: for example, if you were to lie on your back with your knees bent and tried to flatten your lower back into the floor. The opposite of Anterior Rotation.

Postero–lateral

To move backwards and also to the side. The typical position a prolapsed disc tends to take.

Rotation

Twisting or turning to one side.

Side Flexion

Side-bending your body to one side, as if sliding your arm down the side of one leg.

Unilateral

Applying to one side only, i.e. the left or the right.

THE SPINE/VERTEBRAL COLUMN

The spine (or vertebral column as it is also called) consists of 24 individual vertebrae: 7 Cervical (neck), 12 Thoracic (mid-back) and 5 Lumbar (low back). There also follow 9 fused vertebrae (5 Sacral and 4 Coccygeal).

Looking at the spine from the side, you can see there are three main curves (not including those at the Sacrum and Coccyx region). These curves in the spine are referred to as Lordosis (Cervical and Lumbar region) and Kyphosis (Thoracic region). However, when we look at the spine from behind, you can see how the spine should be straight.

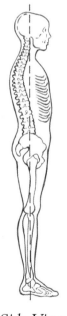

Side View

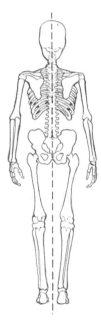

Posterior View

These vertebrae are broken down into their anatomical regions and are often described as:

C1-C7: The 7 vertebra of the Cervical Spine (neck).
T1-T12: The 12 vertebra of the Thoracic Spine (mid-back).
L1-L5: The 5 Vertebra of the Lumbar Spine (lower back).
S1-S5: The 5 fused vertebra of the Sacrum.

Our concern for this book is primarily with the Lumbar Spine and the Sacro-Iliac Joint (SIJ). It is important to note that these do not function independently of the rest of the spine, and this will be considered throughout the book. However, for the purposes of anatomy, explanations confined primarily to the lumbar spine and SIJ will be sufficient.

When looking at the spine from the side and behind as seen on the opposite page, you can see the position the spine should be in. This posture is what I shall refer to as your 'neutral spine'. One of the main contributing factors to low back pain and sciatica, be it caused or maintained by, is prolonged or repeated deviations from this posture. It is imperative for you to aim for this neutral posture as much as is practical if you are to provide your spine with as few inappropriate stresses as possible. This will create the optimum conditions for your body to heal itself.

Lumbar Spine and Sacrum

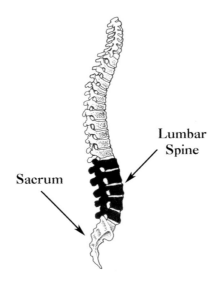

Lumbar
Spine

Sacrum

At the bottom of the spine are the 5 Lumbar Vertebrae, of which the bottom fifth vertebra (L5) articulates with the top of the Sacrum (S1).

Sacro-Iliac Joint

To form the pelvis there are two innominate bones on either side of the Sacrum, which themselves are divided into three anatomical regions. The part of the innominate bone which attaches to the Sacrum is referred to as the Ilium (plural: Ilia). Consequently, these two bones form the Sacro-Iliac joint. There is very little movement that takes place at this joint. However, it can be a source of low back pain.

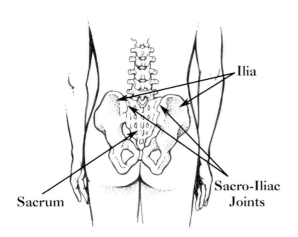

Vertebra

Looking at each individual Vertebra of the spine from above, as shown to the right, you can see the Vertebral Body upon which the disc sits. Just posterior to this is the Vertebral Canal, through which the spinal cord passes (the spinal cord is like a cable of nerves that originate from the brain and pass down through the vertebral canal to the lower part of the spine).

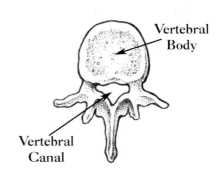

The image below shows how the Vertebra stack upon each other, separated by the Intervertebral Discs.

Vertebra

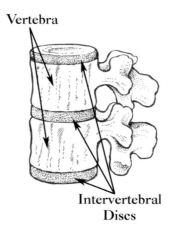

Intervertebral Discs

Facet Joints

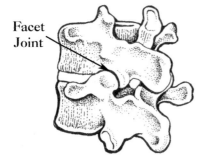

Facet Joint

At the posterior aspect of each vertebra there is an articular surface. This surface articulates with its corresponding surface on the vertebrae below, forming a facet joint. If there is too much pressure placed upon these structures, they can be a source of pain.

Ligaments

The ligaments of the spine, along with the muscles and bony anatomy, provide increased stability for the lower back. This helps prevent increased movement beyond its natural range, which can lead to pain. With regard to the lumbar spine, the ligaments run along the front, back and sides of the vertebra.

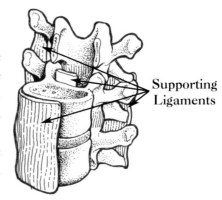

Supporting Ligaments

Nerve Roots

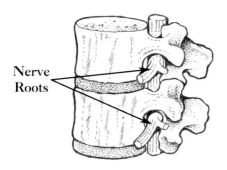

Nerve Roots

As the spinal cord passes down the vertebral canal of the spine, it gives rise to nerve roots at each individual vertebral level. The name of the nerve root is dictated by where it leaves the spinal column. With regard to the lumbar spine, the nerve root is named after the vertebra which it is positioned below. For example, the nerve root between the first (L1) and second (L2) vertebra, is referred to as the L1 nerve root. These nerve roots combine with other nerve roots that in turn form peripheral nerves.

Peripheral Nerves

It is the peripheral nerves which pass all over the body, from the top of our head to the tips of our toes. These enable us to move our muscles and also touch and feel things, including pain. For the purpose of this book we are primarily concerned with the nerve roots of the Lumbar Spine and Sacrum, and in particular L4–S3, which form the *sciatic nerve*. There are other nerves which can contribute to low back and leg pain, but it tends to be the sciatic nerve which is the main culprit.

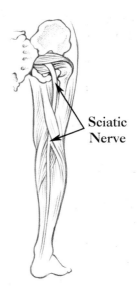

Sciatic Nerve

The sciatic nerve passes deep through the buttock area and into the posterior aspect of the leg towards the knee. It does, however, give rise to other peripheral nerves as it travels further down the leg.

The term 'Sciatica' is only a descriptive and not a diagnostic one. It is given to any pain which is felt in the region of the sciatic nerve. However, there are different causes of sciatica.

Intervertebral Discs

Individual vertebrae of the spine are divided from one another by fibrous intervertebral discs. These help provide mobility and shock absorbency for the spine.

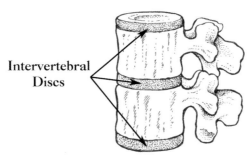

Intervertebral
Discs

If you were to view the vertebra from above, you would see how the disc sits upon the vertebral body. These discs have an inner soft jelly-like core, known as the *Nucleus Pulposus*, and a stronger outer fibrous layer called the *Annulus Fibrosus*.

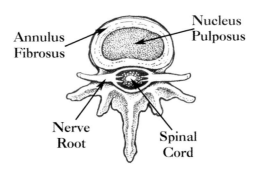

Nucleus
Pulposus

Annulus
Fibrosus

Nerve
Root

Spinal
Cord

It is the *Nucleus Pulposus* that can create a bulging of the disc, which may then lead to pain. When this does occur, it typically bulges in a postero-lateral direction and therefore can compress the nerve root at that particular level.

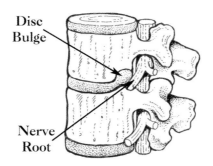

Bulging disc viewed from the side.

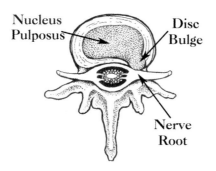

Bulging disc viewed from above.

MUSCLES

The lower back and pelvis are further complemented by groups of muscles that provide mobility and stability to the spine. I will show and describe not only the primary muscles of the lower back, but also other muscles that may not be quite so important with regard to movement, but can play a vital role with regard to causes of low back pain and sciatica, especially if they are tight or weak.

All of the muscles given are drawn with reference to adjacent bones, enabling you to visualise their exact position on the body.

Anterior Muscles

Abdominals

These consist of four muscle groups: Rectus Abdominis, Internal Oblique, External Oblique and Transversus Abdominis.

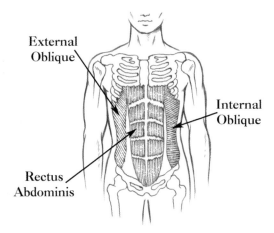

> *Rectus Abdominis:* whose primary role is involved with flexion of the spine (similar to when a sit-up is performed).

> *Internal and External Obliques:* these assist in flexion of the spine when working bilaterally with the Rectus Abdominis, or in rotation of the spine when working unilaterally.

➤ *Transversus Abdominis:* this is an important stabilising muscle of the lower back. This muscle, ***which is situated underneath the Rectus Abdominis, Internal and External Obliques,*** assists in flattening the abdominal wall and strengthening the lower back, therefore helping to maintain a neutral spine.

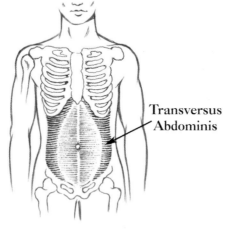

Transversus
Abdominis

ILIOPSOAS

This consists primarily of two muscles, *Iliacus* and *Psoas Major.* Psoas Major is attached to all of the lumbar vertebrae and passes down across the hip joint to attach to the top of the femur (upper leg). The Iliacus muscle attaches to the inside 'lip' of the pelvis and passes down to blend in with the tendon of Psoas Major mentioned above. The main muscle relating to low back pain would be Psoas Major, which can increase lumbar extension when tight.

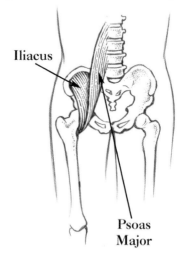

Iliacus

Psoas
Major

This is a group of four muscles that pass down the front of the thigh. The primary muscle here that can influence low back pain is the Rectus Femoris. This is due to this particular muscle attaching to the pelvis and assisting with flexion of the hip. If this is tight, it can create increased anterior rotation of the pelvis, which itself increases lumbar extension. The other three muscles attach to the femur and have the primary role of knee extension.

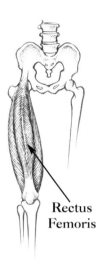

Rectus
Femoris

Posterior Muscles

ERECTOR SPINAE

These are a group of muscles that run along either side of the spine, with their primary function being that of extension if working bilaterally, or side flexion if working unilaterally. This muscle group is shown only on the left-hand side of the drawing below.

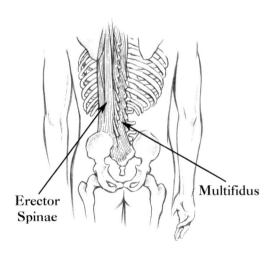

Erector
Spinae

Multifidus

MULTIFIDUS

These are also a group of muscles that run alongside the spine and are positioned 'underneath' the previously mentioned Erector Spinae. Although these muscles are positioned at the back of the spine and are said to assist with extension, their primary role is seen to be that of stabilisation of the spine.

There are insertions from the Multifidi muscles to each lumbar vertebra; consequently they have an extremely important stabilising effect upon each individual vertebra they are attached to. These muscles are shown only on the right-hand side of the drawing at the bottom of the opposite page, where the more superficial Erector Spinae muscles have been 'removed'.

PIRIFORMIS

This muscle is situated deep within the buttock region, is attached to the sacrum and passes down and outwards to attach to the Greater Trochanter of the femur. With regard to this muscle's action, it can be a little confusing as it depends upon the position of the hip. It externally rotates the hip when the hip is flexed no more than approximately 60 degrees and internally rotates when the hip is flexed more than approximately 60 degrees. In my experience, I would say this muscle being tight is one of the main causes/ maintainers of low-back pain and sciatica.

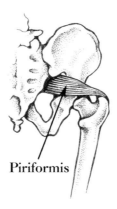

Piriformis

GLUTEALS

A powerful muscle group, essential for movement and stability during activities such as walking and running. This group consists of the large Gluteus Maximus, whose primary action is hip extension and then the smaller Gluteus Medius and Gluteus Minimus muscles, which are involved in abduction of the hip.

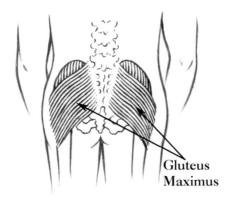

Gluteus
Maximus

HAMSTRINGS

A group of three muscles on the posterior aspect of the thigh. These muscles have an action over two joints, the hip and the knee. This book is mainly concerned with its influence over the hip and consequently the pelvis, to which it is attached. This group of muscles assist with extension of the hip. If tight, they can encourage a posterior rotation of the pelvis, which in turn will tend to flex the lumbar spine.

Hamstrings

Latissimus Dorsi

This is a very large muscle, travelling from the upper part of the arm down towards the pelvis. With regard to the lower back, when working bilaterally this muscle has an action of tilting the pelvis anteriorly, which contributes to extension of the lumbar spine. If working unilaterally it will assist in side flexion of the spine.

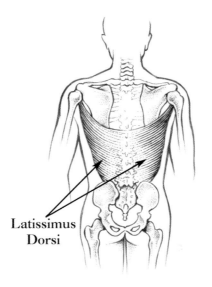

Latissimus Dorsi

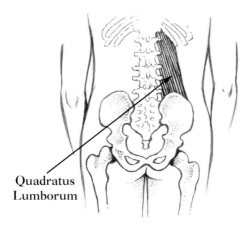

Quadratus Lumborum

Quadratus Lumborum

This muscle is positioned either side of the lumbar spine, although it is only shown on the right side in the given diagram. It helps assist with lumbar extension when working on both sides of the spine or side bending when working unilaterally.

GASTROCNEMIUS

The Gastrocnemius muscle is the larger of the two calf muscles and attaches to just above the knee and then blends in to form the Achilles tendon at the back of the ankle.

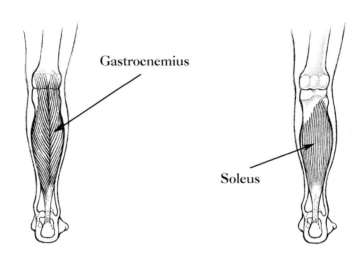

SOLEUS

The Soleus muscle is the smaller of the two calf muscles and is situated underneath the large Gastrocnemius muscle. Soleus attaches just below the knee and then travels down to form the Achilles tendon along with the Gastrocnemius muscle.

Although the Gastrocnemius and Soleus muscles do not really have a significant influence over low back pain and sciatica as such, it is not unusual for those suffering with sciatica to have pain and tightness in the calf region. If this is the case, it is important that the nerves that pass through this area are as supple and mobile as possible. Consequently, if these muscles are tight, they may be restricting the nerves a little, thereby contributing to any pain and discomfort being felt.

Inner Thigh

ADDUCTORS

These muscles pass from the pelvis down and along the inside of the thigh, performing the function of pulling your leg towards the mid-line when contracting, i.e. Adduction.

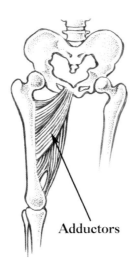

Adductors

That completes what I feel is the functional anatomy of the lower back and pelvis. I would say you have just read all that, and probably more than you need know in order to begin curing yourself of your pain. Remember, there is no need to memorise this chapter, just flick back if you feel you need to.

The chapter **Learning Zone: *Why You are Feeling Pain*** follows, which will give you an understanding of why your lower back can end up causing you so much pain and also of the different types of pain you may be experiencing.

Learning Zone:

Why You are Feeling Pain

As you now have an understanding of the functional anatomy of the lower back, pelvis and sciatic nerve, this chapter will explain why I believe most people suffer with low back pain and sciatica. In addition to this, I will explain the different types of pain, namely, inflammatory and mechanical, from which you are likely to be suffering.

The lower back, like the whole body, has to deal with numerous stresses during our day-to-day activities. These are stresses that the body usually tolerates with no problems whatsoever. However, like everything in life, our back has a threshold level (in this case relative to pain) and once this level has been breached we experience pain.

I'm going to use the first of many analogies here simply to highlight this point. Let's say we tie some string to a wall in our house and every time we walk past it we give it a few firm tugs. For the first few times it is unlikely anything significant will happen. However, as we repeat this many times, it is likely that somewhere along the length of the string some of the individual strands will begin to give. As we continue to repeat pulling on the string, it will eventually fray significantly and ultimately tear or snap.

Now I'm not saying that your back is going to tear or snap in any way: it will not. I have used this example to highlight that the string is able to tolerate the stresses being placed upon it initially, but eventually the cumulative effect of these stresses will begin to tell and the string will start to give until it eventually fails.

Exactly the same principle occurs when you place cumulative stresses upon your lower back and associated structures, including the sciatic nerve. The advantage of our body, however, is that as soon as it realises the stresses being placed upon it are accumulating too much, it will let you know by sending pain messages to your brain. This is its warning system that you need to change things, as what you are doing is potentially harming it.

If you heed this warning and ease off or modify the offending activities which are aggravating your low back or sciatic nerve, the stresses across your back will subside. Any minor damage which may have taken place will be repaired by the body and therefore any pain you were suffering will also be resolved.

However, if you ignore this warning, these same stresses will continue to accumulate. As the stresses across your back increase, your body's warning system will become more noticeable and you will experience increased pain.

This cycle of increased stress leading to increased pain will continue until you begin to address and reduce the stresses which are causing the pain. When you do this, the body will once again begin to heal itself and therefore the pain will begin to subside.

If you do not ease off, however, this cycle of increasing pain will continue until eventually you have no choice but to modify things, as the pain will be too intense. Your body will win in the end. If it needs you to reduce the stresses you are placing upon it in order to heal itself, and you are not listening to its warnings, it will in effect force you to do so by increasing the pain to an intolerable level.

I'm sure you are familiar with this scenario, be it with your current pain, where maybe you are unable to even put your socks on, or maybe another injury, let's say to your ankle.

With this latter example of ankle pain, immediately after the injury you may only be able to place a very small, if any, amount of weight on your ankle due to increased pain. This is because the body is telling you to rest the injured area while it works away at healing itself. Any more than that would increase the pain levels and therefore be hindering the body's own healing process.

If you were to ignore this and still try to place excess weight on your ankle, you know the pain levels would increase until it is simply too painful to place any weight whatsoever on it.

If, however, you listen to your body and place decreased stresses on your injured ankle, you also know the body will gradually begin to heal itself and the pain will therefore decrease. As the levels of pain decrease, you will find you can begin to place more and more stress on your ankle, until eventually you will have no problem in placing your full weight on it.

This is a typical example of your body generating increased pain in response to an injury, with the result that you decrease the amount of stress being placed on it. As you decrease the stresses, the body will begin to heal itself and the structures involved will heal and become stronger and the pain will consequently disappear.

I will not labour this point any more here, as it will be covered in more detail in **Step Three: *How to Optimising Your Body's Healing Potential.*** I have just outlined it here to show why we experience pain and how our perception of pain will increase if we do not heed our body's warning system.

It is my belief that these continued stresses placed upon the lower back and sciatic nerve which lead to pain, are a result of incorrect postures and movement patterns along with muscle imbalance. These two go very much hand in hand.

INCORRECT POSTURES & MOVEMENT PATTERNS

Your body is truly amazing with regard to what it is capable of. During our day-to-day activities we move around, stand and sit without even thinking about it, as the body naturally tells us how to do so. Unfortunately though, as we do so thousands and thousands of times, we can subtly learn incorrect ways of performing these day-to-day activities.

NB. The terms I am about to use now, FDP and EDP, stand for Flexion Dominated Pain and Extension Dominated Pain respectively. These terms will be fully explained during **Step Four: *How to Diagnose Your Pain*.** If you wish to learn about these terms first, simply flick forward to this chapter. However, it is not essential for you to understand them at this stage, so feel free to read on.

Incorrect Postures

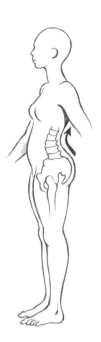

A **postural** example I am going to use is standing. I have seen many people attend the physiotherapy department who have developed a poor posture in standing, and it is this that is contributing to their pain. Typically, this tends to be where the natural lordotic arch in the lower back is increased. This usually results in the patient having a functional diagnosis of Extension Dominated Pain (EDP).

Incorrect Movement Patterns

The **movement** example I am going to use is that of bending, a very common one which I am sure you are aware of. Far too many of us, when bending forward, keep our hips and knees fairly straight and use the back for nearly all of the movement (see the diagram below left).

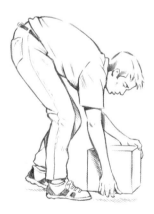

This places far too much stress upon the spine and in particular the posterior aspect of the lower back and its discs. This incorrect movement pattern would usually result in the patient concerned developing Flexion Dominated Pain (FDP).

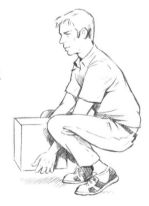

I'm sure you know the correct way to lift is using your hips and knees (as shown in the diagram on the bottom right of the opposite page). If you do not, an easy way to find out is to either watch yourself now or observe someone lifting with a painful back. It will be very rare, if at all, that you will see someone with a bad back lifting like the person in the picture as shown in the diagram on the bottom left of the opposite page. The person with the bad back will tend to lift using their hips and knees a little more and keep their back as straight as possible. This is because they know it will cause them less pain. It will cause them less pain because it places less stress across the back and therefore encourages the healing process to take place. This is the fundamental principle used throughout this book.

As I mentioned, the examples I have given for incorrect postural and movement patterns will be elaborated on fully as you progress through this book, in particular during the chapter, **Learning Zone:** *Why Muscles are the Key Factor in Eliminating Your Pain.*

MUSCLE IMBALANCE

This refers to the different muscle groups that work together to provide our body with movement and stability. If any of these muscles are particularly tight or weak, they can place increased stresses upon the structures they have an influence over.

If muscles are too tight, they will 'pull' or 'tug' on the structures they are attached to. For example, tight Hamstrings can encourage increased posterior rotation of the pelvis, which may relatively increase flexion of the lower back. They can also place increased stress upon the sciatic nerve as the latter passes through them.

If muscles are too weak however, they will not be able to exert enough stability across the structures they are designed to support; incorrect movement patterns may therefore occur. For example, weak abdominals will find it difficult to maintain the neutral position of the lower back, typically resulting in anterior rotation of the pelvis and subsequent extension of the lumbar spine.

If I can just reinforce what I have mentioned before, there is no need to understand these examples fully. You will gain a more thorough understanding as you read through this book, in particular during the chapter **Learning Zone:** *Why Muscles are the Key Factor in Eliminating Your Pain*.

These two concepts – of incorrect postures and movement patterns, and muscle imbalance – go hand in hand because one can lead to the other.

If you adopt incorrect postures as you go about your day-to-day activities, you will be using your muscles incorrectly. This in turn can result in some muscles becoming weak and others becoming tight. Alternatively, if you have specific tight or weak muscles, this may result in you developing incorrect postures and movement patterns as the muscles are unable to 'hold' or 'move' you the correct way.

This in itself can create a 'chicken and egg' scenario with regard to which came first. Either way, a vicious cycle often results where they reinforce each other. The aim of this book is to provide you with the knowledge in order to identify first any of these potential causes of pain and then, with the appropriate advice and exercises, eliminate them.

This will result in a positive cycle whereby correct postures and movements encourage the muscles to work appropriately. With the muscles working as they should, the weak ones will become stronger and the tight ones will become supple. With them being stronger and more supple, they will be able to work more efficiently, therefore encouraging correct posture and movements…and so on.

TYPES OF PAIN

So we have now established there are primarily two main reasons why you may suffer from low back pain or sciatica, incorrect postures and movement patterns, and muscle imbalance. I shall now move on to explain the two different types of pain you are likely to experience.

It is important I highlight here, however, that nothing is black and white as far as the human body is concerned. There is without doubt a great deal of overlap with the following types of pain. These two types of pain can also 'work together' as is described towards the end of this chapter, which deals with 'acute on chronic' pain. However, for ease of explanation, they have been described separately.

Acute / Inflammatory Pain

With this type of pain, the pain threshold level may have been breached as a result of a traumatic event, e.g. a fall or road traffic accident. Or, perhaps, as a result of multiple micro-trauma, e.g. repeated bending or lifting.

> *With regard to the latter micro-trauma example, I have had many patients say to me they were only doing up their shoelaces / putting their socks on / picking something up, etc. when their back 'went'. The problem here is it is likely to be the hundreds, probably thousands, of times they have performed that action before that has contributed towards the pain. This last time, to coin a phrase, is 'the straw that broke the camel's back'.*

The problem that now arises is that this 'injury' is likely to have set up an inflammatory response. The chemicals produced by this inflammatory response will stimulate the pain nerve fibres, which themselves send messages to the brain screaming **PAIN!** This pain is likely to be ***severe, constant and unremitting, and relief from this type of pain seems practically impossible.***

However, not only do the inflammatory chemicals stimulate the receptors of the pain nerve fibres, but they also sensitise them, making them more readily stimulated to send further pain messages to the brain. This results in a vicious cycle, whereby the inflammation present decreases the threshold levels of pain. Therefore even the slightest of pressures or smallest of activities about the area concerned results in increased pain perception and the area becoming further aggravated and inflamed. This increased inflammation means the pain threshold levels will be decreased once again and therefore the injured area will become more painful as it is more readily aggravated, resulting in increased inflammation and so on.

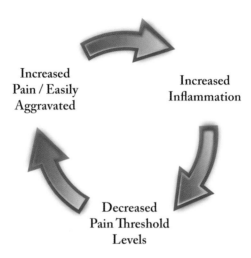

Increased
Pain / Easily
Aggravated

Increased
Inflammation

Decreased
Pain Threshold
Levels

I often use the analogy here of hitting your thumb with a hammer. You only have to do this once, but you can bet your life for the next few days you only have to brush your thumb against something and the thumb will start to throb and ache yet again, becoming even more sensitive. This is the body's way of telling you to stop aggravating it while it is trying to heal itself. As you avoid aggravating it though, the sensitivity and pain will gradually settle until you feel no pain at all.

The primary aim of treatment at this stage is to settle the inflammatory response and therefore decrease the sensitivity present. With regard to your low back pain and sciatica, this will be covered in **Step Two:** *How to STOP Acutely Inflamed Pain*.

Mechanical Pain

This type of pain presents as what I tend to refer to as an 'on/off' pain, i.e. if you put yourself in a certain position or perform a certain activity, you feel pain, yet if you remove yourself from that particular position or activity, the pain goes away. It is also the classic grumbling, nagging pain that has usually been around for some time, many months or even years.

This doesn't tend to be as debilitating as the acute inflammatory pain, in that it doesn't give you a constant, often vicious, striking pain which can take your breath away. It tends to be more of a pain about which people often say ***"I have got used to it"*** or ***"I've learned to live with it"***.

In some respects this is like the acute pain, in that there may be a degree of inflammation present. However, I tend to refer to this as low grade inflammation, i.e. not as intense as the inflammatory response set up with acute pain, where everything seems to hurt.

The reason why this mechanical pain often maintains itself is that we subconsciously avoid the stressful postures and activities that originally aggravated it, so as not to increase the pain further. For example, you may avoid any gardening or housework or maybe simply modify how you put your underwear, shoes and socks on in the morning. However, we fail to address all of the stresses which are maintaining this subtly increased sensitivity in the first place.

Therefore the back will heal itself to a certain degree, but not completely as there are still underlying problems preventing the body's healing process from finishing the job. These underlying problems are usually muscle imbalances, which we have previously discussed. However, because these imbalances are not addressed, the pain becomes something that "I just tend to live with".

This is quite simply burying our head in the sand. Although we may be avoiding the aggravating factors in order to prevent the acute inflammatory pain from rearing its ugly head, a fundamental principle used throughout this book, we are doing nothing to address the cause as to why your back is still grumbling away with a nagging type of pain – the one you are just 'learning to live with'.

The aim of treatment here is to discover which stresses upon your back are keeping the pain threshold at a constantly inappropriate low level. If we can discover these stresses and eliminate them accordingly, the pain will once again resolve as the body begins to heal itself.

I would just like to reiterate what I mentioned earlier in this chapter, that the distinction between inflammatory and mechanical pain is not black and white, but rather different shades of grey.

There is no threshold point where the pain turns from primarily inflammatory to primarily mechanical or vice versa. Only you can judge which type of pain you are feeling. A good rule of thumb however is:

Acute/Inflammatory Pain: This tends to be constant and easily aggravated, i.e. you may carry out a quite simple activity/posture and you will feel a sharp 'stab' of pain and/or the throbbing and aching increases. You also know it will probably take some time to settle down. This pain responds well to anti-inflammatories.

Chronic/Mechanical Pain: This tends to be more like a pain you can turn on and off by changing your posture or activity. This type of pain doesn't respond as well to anti-inflammatories.

Acute on Chronic Pain

If you have had your low back pain or sciatica for some time, with it being primarily mechanical in nature, we often refer to it as being a 'chronic' pain problem. When we talk about an attack of pain as being 'acute on chronic' all we are referring to is that the individual concerned has been suffering with mechanical pain for some time, i.e. chronic. However, as a result of the cause of this mechanical pain not being addressed, the constant stresses placed across the lower back will mean the threshold level for an acute attack of pain is never too far away. Consequently, from time to time, an acute inflammatory episode of pain will occur.

The individual concerned thinks he or she knows how to treat this. A couple of days off work or 'taking it easy' is usually enough for the back to return to its normal self, i.e. the grumbling old chronic pain which he/

she has learned to live with. The problem here is that these continuous stresses plus acute episodes of pain are driving the threshold levels further down.

The typical pattern that then results is one where the acute episodes of pain are more intense and last longer, with the periods of relief gained in between becoming shorter and shorter. Without even noticing it, the normal level of low back pain or sciatica the individual has learned to live with subtly increases in intensity and eventually a constant debilitating problem results.

SO HOW DO WE STOP THIS?

We simply have to let the body heal itself...

Easier said than done? No, not really, as long as we give the body the right conditions to heal itself. Whenever we develop acute pain, we automatically avoid the aggravating factors, as we know if we do not the pain will increase substantially. The problem is that we do not really think about why we are doing this. I hope that you now realise why.

One reason is to avoid traumatising the structures concerned further and therefore causing more pain. However, equally, if not more importantly, is that we do this to avoid interfering with the healing process. What we need to do now is continue with this principle in a structured manner so the body can continue to heal itself 100 per cent, rather than to a point where the pain settles to a level "*I can live with*".

> *If you heed the advice given throughout this book, you will enable your body to heal itself completely and therefore you will begin to lead a life free of low back pain/sciatica.*

This is where the following chapter, **Learning Zone:** *Your Own Body is the Greatest Healer* will help explain things further. It will highlight why I believe we all have access to the greatest healer of all – ourselves. If we provide our body with the correct environment it will, without doubt, begin to heal itself. There is no reason why this shouldn't be to the point where you become 100 per cent pain-free and are therefore able to enjoy all the activities you used to before you developed your current episode of pain.

Learning Zone:

Your Own Body is the Greatest Healer

The chapter you are about to read is probably the most important and fundamental way in which you are going to free yourself of pain. No fancy manipulative techniques or flashing lights on electrotherapy equipment. I am going to explain very simply how, if given the correct environment and conditions, your own body will heal itself of the pain you are suffering.

Ultimately, there is only one healer and that is the body itself. Even when surgeons perform fantastic surgery to save or improve the quality of someone's life, they still rely on the body's healing process to complete the task in hand by repairing the trauma caused by the disease/injury itself, as well as repairing the trauma caused by the surgery, i.e. the incisions made to carry out the surgery.

So where does the body go wrong with low back pain and sciatica?

The answer to this question is that the body doesn't go wrong, it will continuously strive to heal itself twenty-four hours a day, seven days a week. The problem lies within ourselves in that we do not always give the body the correct conditions to heal itself; in effect, we keep interfering with our body's own healing process.

I am always using this simple analogy to highlight this point. Let's say we have just cut ourselves. The process which follows is bleeding, which then gradually forms a weak scab and as time passes this scab becomes stronger and stronger while the body slowly replaces the scab itself with scar tissue – the body's wonderful healing process in action.

Now let's imagine that as soon as this scab begins to form we keep on rubbing, scratching and picking it. We all know what will happen, the cut will start bleeding again in order to form a new scab. If we keep on picking and scratching it, this process will continue back and forth, i.e. the body trying to heal itself by forming a scab as we interfere with the healing process by the continued agitation of the wound. We are quite obviously interfering with the body's healing process.

Does the body give up? NO, of course it doesn't, it continues relentlessly to heal itself and as soon as we stop interfering with it for long enough, the healing process will be completed. This is why a wound across your elbow or one of your finger joints seems to take a lot longer to heal, due to the bending of that joint continuously interfering with the healing process.

Well, a similar thing happens when we have low back pain or sciatica, although not quite as dramatically as the open wound and significant bleeding a cut produces. If for whatever reason our lower back/sciatic nerve is injured, the body will once again strive to heal itself.

However, if we continue to stress those structures that are trying to heal themselves, it is the equivalent of scratching or picking a scab, in that the healing process is interfered with. Therefore, at best, the traumatised structures will take a lot longer to heal – at worst, the pain will continue to increase.

The beauty of the human body is that it does not give up! If we reverse this situation by not only taking these stresses away from the injured structures, but also provide them with the optimum healing conditions, *the body will heal itself and your pain will be resolved*.

This is what this book is all about, providing you with the appropriate advice and exercises so as to enable your body's own healing process to cure itself of pain. As you continue reading, you will learn how to provide yourself with a functional diagnosis for your pain. You will then go on to gain the knowledge that relates to how to take the inappropriate stresses away from your lower back and/or sciatic nerve in order for it to heal itself; at the same time you will also learn how to place the appropriate stresses upon those same structures in order for them to become stronger. This in turn will *allow you to carry out all of the activities you were doing before you had any low back pain or sciatica.*

I promise you that sometimes it really can be that simple. If you give your body the appropriate conditions, it will heal itself.

I have treated patients before who have suffered with low back pain or sciatica for many years. They then made a few simple alterations to the way in which they carry out certain activities and their pain fully resolved itself. Now I am not going to say it is always that straightforward, but it can be…

If you give your body the appropriate conditions, it will heal itself.

The following chapter **Step Two: *How to STOP Acutely Inflamed Pain*** will show you how to calm down the intense pain suffered by someone with an acute attack of low back pain or sciatica. Some of the positions you are asked to adopt during that chapter will make reference to FDP (Flexion Dominated Pain) and EDP (Extension Dominated Pain).

Although I have yet to discuss the concept of FDP and EDP, it will be covered in great detail throughout this book, particularly during **Step Four: *How to Diagnose Your Pain***.

The reason I have put the following chapter in before these diagnostic terms have been explained is because it is vitally important we try to resolve the intense pain and sensitivity felt when suffering with acutely inflamed pain as soon as possible.

When you are suffering with pain that is sensitive and intolerable, we really do have our hands tied with regard to you performing the specific exercises I would wish you to in order to resolve your pain completely. Therefore, if we can settle this sensitivity down as soon as possible, we will then progress quickly towards the more specific exercises you need to perform for your particular functional diagnosis.

Step Two:

How to STOP Acutely Inflamed Pain

If you are reading this book now and suffering with acutely inflamed pain, this chapter will show you how to best resolve this as soon as possible, enabling you to move on and provide yourself with a *self-prescribed exercise programme* to resolve your pain completely.

You will now have a good understanding of the functional anatomy of the lower back, why we all tend to develop low back pain and sciatica, the different types of pain we may experience and how fantastic the body's healing process is.

As you use this chapter to help resolve your acutely inflamed pain, that pain will become more mechanical in its nature and therefore less sensitive. With it being less sensitive, you will be able to progress further into the different types of exercises to be performed, all of which are covered in great detail in the subsequent chapters.

I would just like to reiterate what I said at the end of the previous chapter. While reading the following, you will find reference to FDP (Flexion Dominated Pain) and EDP (Extension Dominated Pain). Do not be put off if you do not understand what they mean, as I have yet to explain their definitions and how they may relate to your pain. The reason they are mentioned here is to give you further understanding as to why certain positions may help specific diagnoses, one of which you will be suffering from.

All will become clear as you read through this book. If you are feeling impatient and would like to have a grasp of these terms before you read this chapter, just move on to **Step Four:** *How to Diagnose Your Pain* where you will soon become familiar with this terminology. I have placed this chapter here simply because if you are suffering with acutely inflamed pain, we need to address this as soon as we can.

INFLAMMATORY BACK PAIN

This type of pain presents itself typically as the acute inflammatory pain described in the earlier chapter, **Learning Zone:** *Why You are Feeling Pain*. This is where the pain is pretty much unremitting and very easily aggravated. This, without doubt, can be the most debilitating of pains. The first and most obvious thing to do with this type of pain is to decrease the inflammatory response taking place.

There are two main ways you can reduce this inflammatory response, either by taking some anti-inflammatories or stop aggravating it:

Anti-inflammatories

I know this may be a slightly contentious issue, considering press reports about the possible side effects some anti-inflammatories may have on people with heart conditions. However, on the whole they are safe to take.

If you do suffer with any kind of heart condition, asthma, stomach problems or if you are taking regular medication or feel you may not be able to take anti-inflammatories for whatever reason, it is important to speak to your GP regarding this matter first.

If it is okay for you to take anti-inflammatories, it is important to take them regularly. I have treated many patients who take anti-inflammatories on a 'when I need to' basis, but this is not the best way to take them. Let me explain first the principle difference between painkillers and anti-inflammatories with regard to pain.

If you are in pain and have an inflammatory response taking place, the body is producing inflammatory chemicals that themselves stimulate pain nerve fibres. It is these pain nerve fibres that send the pain messages to the brain and results in you feeling your pain. The main difference between pain killers and anti-inflammatories lies in whereabouts in the body they have their effect on preventing you from feeling pain.

With regard to ***pain killers***, these simply prevent the pain messages from being perceived by your brain. If this message is stopped, you will feel no pain. However, with ***anti-inflammatories,*** they stop or reduce the inflammatory response taking place. As a result of this, there are no harsh chemicals present to stimulate the pain nerve fibres in the first place. If these pain fibres are not being stimulated, they are unable to send pain messages to the brain, therefore there is no pain.

In effect, the anti-inflammatories are addressing the main cause of the pain, i.e. the cause of the pain nerve fibres being stimulated. However, ultimately we need to find and address the cause of the inflammation itself. This book will set out to achieve this as soon as the acute inflammatory phase has been dealt with.

The best way to take painkillers is to take them in an 'on demand' manner, i.e. when you have pain. With regard to anti-inflammatories, however, it is best to have them in your system twenty-four hours a day, consistently mopping up all of the inflammatory chemicals as they are produced.

It is important I stress here that you will not be taking the anti-inflammatories in order to mask the pain. I would never advocate that. You will be taking them as a means to an end. By taking the anti-inflammatories regularly, you will be constantly reducing the sensitivity of your pain, which itself will mean the pain is not as easily aggravated.

If your pain is not as easily aggravated, you will be able to perform the appropriate exercises more readily in order to stretch and strengthen the structures concerned, without interfering with the healing process. Finally, as the structures concerned become more supple and stronger, the pain you are suffering will naturally be resolved and therefore you can start to reduce the medication you are taking.

TAKING MEDICATION

*If you are in any doubt as to whether you are able to take certain medication, it is important you discuss this with your GP/health professional first. Also, if you suffer **any side effects at all** with regard to taking anti-inflammatories, it is important to stop taking them immediately and speak to your GP.*

A typical complaint with regard to anti-inflammatories is that they can upset the stomach. If this does occur, it may be okay to take a different type or lower dose anti-inflammatory. Once again, discuss this with your GP.

> *Anti-inflammatories can also exacerbate the signs and symptoms associated with asthma. Therefore, if you suffer with asthma, no matter how mild, do not take anti-inflammatories without first discussing this matter with your GP.*

One final thing, you should definitely notice a significant improvement within a week or so, probably much sooner, as a result of taking anti-inflammatories. If you do not, they are not working for you.

If you are still convinced your pain is inflammatory in nature, I suggest you speak to your GP with regard to either:

i) Trying some stronger anti-inflammatories.
ii) Trying a different type of anti-inflammatory, as some people respond better to different types and you may need to change the ones you are taking.

If they still have no effect on your pain, you may as well stop taking them as they are obviously not working.

I am like most people in that I try to avoid taking medication as much as possible. However, I have seen enough people suffering with pain to know that sometimes medication is required. Nevertheless, if you are taking medication and it is not helping you, what's the point in taking it! This may seem obvious, but I have treated many patients who have been prescribed anti-inflammatories by their GP for months on end and they are still taking them even though they are not helping.

Do not automatically think anti-inflammatories will not work for you if you have taken them before with little success. I have treated many patients who have said this to me, yet the reason they did not help was because they continued to perform their aggravating activities. Although anti-inflammatories can be a great way of reducing inflammation, they are not a 'magic bullet'. If you continue to aggravate your pain at a greater rate than which the anti-inflammatories can resolve the inflammation, the painful inflammatory response is going to win. At best, your pain will feel better while on the anti-inflammatories, yet it will simply return as soon as you stop taking them.

In addition to this, people sometimes have taken anti-inflammatories on a 'when I need to' basis as opposed to how they are prescribed. As I have mentioned, this is not an appropriate way to take them and if you were taking them like this I would suggest you try another course to see how they work, only this time take them regularly.

As I have already stated, I am not suggesting you take this form of medication in order to mask the pain, definitely not. I am asking you to take these in addition to providing your body with the appropriate conditions to heal itself. By doing this, it will help you break through the vicious cycle often created by inflammation and therefore help speed up your body's healing process.

Stop aggravating it

I tend to refer to this as 'nature's way'. If you stop aggravating an inflamed structure, there is every chance it will resolve itself, thanks to the wonderful healing process of the human body. This was discussed in the earlier chapter, **Learning Zone: *Why You are Feeling Pain.***

The analogy given in that particular chapter, with regard to hitting your thumb with a hammer, is a very good one. It shows how a very acutely inflamed structure, i.e. the thumb, can so easily be aggravated, yet will resolve itself given the correct conditions.

Well, this scenario applies to any structure in the human body, not just the thumb. Therefore your low back pain or sciatica can also be resolved of any inflammatory response present if you give it a chance.

However, in the early stages of acute pain there may be no position or activity which completely alleviates it. In such circumstances, we just need to find the most pain-relieving position we can, i.e. the one that keeps your pain down to a minimum.

Some typical positions are as follows:

1) *Side Lying with pillows*

2) *Prone Lying with pillows*

3) *Prone Lying*

4) *Crook Lying*

5) *Lying with your feet supported on a chair*

With regard to these positions, I will highlight which, as a rule of thumb, will best suit the type of pain you may be suffering with. At this stage a functional diagnosis is not important, as the immediate aim is to reduce the acute inflammatory response taking place. Therefore, simply find the most comfortable position you can for your pain. **Step Four:** ***How to Diagnose Your Pain*** *will explain how you can determine which functional diagnosis it is you are suffering with. Feel free to advance to this chapter now if you wish to familiarise yourself with this terminology, but it is not essential at this stage.*

1) SIDE LYING WITH PILLOWS

This position tends to be best if you lie on one side, have your bottom leg straight and place the top leg on a couple of pillows. This is a good neutral position, in that by keeping the bottom leg straight it helps keep the lower back in a neutral position. Also by keeping the top leg supported by pillows, it prevents this leg from 'rolling forwards and down' which itself can create a twisting motion upon the lower back and therefore be painful.

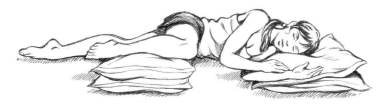

If your pain is incredibly intense and irritable, regardless of what you feel your diagnosis is, Side Lying with pillows is usually the most comfortable position of the five given in this chapter.

2) Prone Lying with Pillows and 3) Prone Lying

These two are generally better for the person suffering with FDP. If your pain is particularly intense, lying on your stomach may be too painful. If this is the case, try lying with one or two pillows under your stomach, as you will probably find this more comfortable.

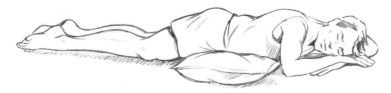

As the pain begins to settle, gradually reduce the number of pillows you are lying on, until eventually you are just lying flat on your stomach.

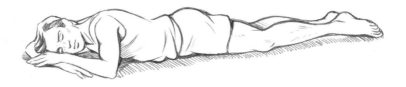

4) Crook Lying and 5) Lying with your feet supported on a chair

These are typically more suited for the individual suffering with EDP. It is particularly important to have the hips bent, as if you are suffering with EDP you may also have tight hip flexor muscles and therefore lying with your legs out straight may aggravate your pain – see Quadriceps & Psoas in the chapter, **Learning Zone: *Why Muscles are the Key Factor in Eliminating Your Pain.***

Whether you are in Crook Lying or Lying with your feet supported on a chair, by keeping your hips in this bent position, it will help reduce the pressure placed upon your lower back by the pull of the tight hip flexor muscles.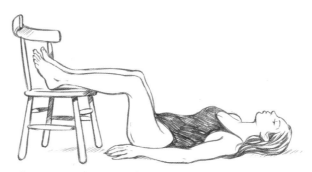

Whichever of the previous five positions you find the most comfortable, *I would ask you to adopt this position for about five minutes at least every hour.* As always, nothing I suggest in this book is set in stone. If you carry out such positions and you feel it aggravates your pain, it is important to ease off.

The reason I say ease off, and not stop, is because it may be the right position for you to adopt; it's just that you may be doing a bit too much too soon. If you have eased off a few times and it still aggravates your pain, then modify this position or simply stop using it and look for a more suitable one.

Of equal importance though, is that if you adopt such a position and you feel it really helps, feel free to do it more often or for longer. You will find as you read through this book that I am a great believer in everyone listening to their own body.

If you are aggravating your pain, you are interfering with the healing process, therefore you need to avoid or modify what it is you are doing. On the other hand, if you are carrying out an activity or are in a certain posture that is easing your pain, you will be providing your body with the ideal conditions for healing to take place; therefore I want you to encourage this activity.

In summary, with regard to the positions suggested in this section:

If they ease your pain, encourage them.
If they aggravate your pain, modify or avoid them.

I appreciate that adopting any of these positions on an hourly basis may not always be practical, especially if you are working. Nevertheless, I would like you to aim for this as much as is possible. If you aim for this but are unable to achieve it, then fair enough, but try to avoid simply saying to yourself "that's not possible" as the likelihood then is you will do it very little, if at all.

Ultimately, listen to your pain. The best position in which to place yourself is the one that provides you with most relief. Your body will soon tell you if you are in a position it doesn't like...it will increase your levels of pain.

What about rest?

It is a common misconception that when you have low back pain or sciatica you need to rest it for weeks on end. However, it is equally important not to be misled in the sense that you need to keep active all the time.

*I have treated some patients who have been told by their GP it is important they do not rest their back, they must keep active. I understand why this has been said, but it is also important to be sensible as well. I remember one lady in particular who took a 'No Pain-No Gain' approach – see the final chapter **Old Wives' Tales** for my views on this – and as a result she was constantly aggravating her pain and therefore interfering with the healing process. When arriving for her first appointment she was in an incredible amount of pain. However, as soon as she started to listen to her body and provide it with relative rest as well as activity, it began to settle down fairly quickly. This was then followed by an appropriate exercise programme and it was not too long at all before she was pain-free.*

If your low back pain or sciatica is of a recent onset, and the pain is intense and unremitting, treat it as you would any other acute injury, e.g. a sprained ankle. It may need complete rest for 24-48 hours. If you can keep active during this time, no matter how little, fantastic. If you cannot, however, do not feel guilty about giving yourself a day or two's rest. Remember, by rest I mean the most comfortable position you can find for yourself; one of the five given in this chapter are usually appropriate, but feel free to try another more comfortable one if you can do so.

After this 24-48 hour period, however, you do need to try and increase your activity. If, after 3-4 days, you still cannot perform any activity at all, it is definitely time to call your GP. You may need stronger medication or further investigations. The majority of low back pain and sciatica needs no further investigations at all; however, in this instance it is still best to have it checked by a health professional.

As your pain begins to resolve, and it will do if you give it appropriate and relative rest, you need to become gradually more and more active, as your pain will allow. Once again, remember that the word active is relative, just as the word rest was.

As always, you need constantly to keep an eye on the activities that aggravate and ease your pain, as these may change as your body heals itself and your back becomes stronger. For example, walking could well be an aggravating factor in this early acute inflammatory stage, but as soon as this stage passes it may well become an easing factor. If this does occur, change your activities as appropriate and begin to incorporate walking in to your daily routine more.

It is also not unusual for your functional diagnosis to change as your body heals itself. Therefore, what presented initially as FDP may well become EDP or vice versa. If this does occur, simply change the exercises you are performing accordingly.

As things progress, you will find the inflammatory pain you were suffering with gradually turns into a mechanical type pain. This is exactly what we are aiming for. When this occurs, it is crucial you continue to do the right things for your back, which will now involve becoming more and more active.

The following chapter, **Step Three:** *How to Optimise Your Body's Healing Potential* will explain the best way of trying to further reduce the pain you are suffering, by continuing to establish the aggravating and easing factors. This will help guide you as to which activities it is best to encourage as you become more active and also those which it is still best to modify or avoid.

Step Three:

How to Optimise
Your Body's Healing Potential

From the outset of this book, my aim has been to make resolving your pain as simple as possible, in order for it to be unintrusive with regard to your day-to-day lifestyle. Now that's not to say you will not have to make some temporary sacrifices, you probably will, but they will pale into insignificance when you become pain-free, and besides, nothing is more intrusive than low back pain or sciatica!

As your pain begins to settle, you will find you are becoming more and more active, even if that means you are only walking around a little in between your 'resting' positions. It is important you now continue to encourage the healing process as best you can. Once again, I'm pleased to inform you that if you wish to continue optimising your body's healing process, you need to continue to *stop aggravating it.*

Just as I emphasised earlier with regard to acutely inflamed pain, if you are aggravating your pain, you are interfering with your body's healing process. However, not only will I now ask you to stop aggravating your pain, but I am also going to ask you to encourage any postures and activities that you feel ease it. This is because if you are easing your pain, you will be creating an environment that your body likes, and you will therefore be optimising the healing process.

AGGRAVATING FACTORS

As I am sure you have gathered by now, I am always quick to sing the praises of the human body, and this chapter further emphasises that belief. We now know it isn't difficult to work out what aggravates your pain, you just listen to your body. If you are aggravating and interfering with the body's healing process, you can almost guarantee you will know about it without even thinking, as your levels of discomfort or pain will increase. These are what we will refer to as the *aggravating factors.*

> *Now it is important to stress here that just because you may be doing something that is causing an increase in your pain, it does not mean you are doing any kind of long-term damage to your lower back or sciatic nerve...definitely not. It is simply the body's way of saying you are placing inappropriate stresses across the structures causing you pain and therefore you are interfering with your body's attempts to heal those structures.*
>
> *Thus, although it is important to remember that this message is for your benefit and you need to listen to it, it is equally important you are not fearful of any pain you may be feeling.*
>
> *A common phrase I often use is that you should* **'respect pain, but not be fearful of it'.**

EASING FACTORS

So how do you know when you are giving your body its optimum healing conditions? Once again, you just listen to your body. Only this time you are listening for a reduction in your pain levels. If you are carrying out an activity, exercise or you are in a certain posture which enables the body to begin healing itself, it will say nothing, as it is too busy healing itself. These are what we will refer to as the *easing factors*.

SO WHAT DO I DO NOW?

The first thing you need to do is make some kind of mental note as to what you feel your 'normal' level of pain is. By normal I mean the level of pain that is around most of the time, or the level of pain that you feel you

'just have to live with'. Once you are familiar with this normal level…
ignore it, as this tells us nothing. We are only interested when your pain
feels particularly better or particularly worse than this normal level.

Why should I ignore my normal levels of pain?

As I have explained, it is the deviations from this normal level of pain that
will enable you to establish your aggravating and easing factors. Therefore,
all I ask you to do is continue with your day as planned and whenever
your pain feels particularly better or particularly worse than normal, stop
and ask yourself:

> *"What am I doing now and what have I been doing over
> the last few hours?"*

The reason you need to ask yourself this is because the chances are it is
something you are doing, or have been doing that your pain has either
liked or disliked.

If you have stopped and asked yourself this question because your pain
has increased, i.e. you are/have been performing an *aggravating factor*, make
a note of what you are doing and have been doing for the last few hours,
avoid or modify those activities as you feel appropriate and then resume
your daily routine.

The next time you feel your pain increasing, ask yourself the same question,
make a note, avoid or modify the activity and continue. You need to continue
doing this until you see some kind of pattern emerge. As soon as you start
thinking something along the lines of:

> *"Oh, it seems to be whenever I do…my pain increases."*

avoid or modify this particular activity or posture for the time being as
much as is practical, as it is interfering with your body's healing process!

Equally important is the need for you to identify the easing factors. Once again, continue with your day as planned and whenever you notice your pain has decreased or disappeared completely, ask yourself again:

"What am I doing now and what have I been doing over the last few hours?"

By now, I'm sure you know why you are asking yourself this, but I'll explain nevertheless. You are asking yourself this question and making a note of it, because your pain is probably feeling better at this time as a result of what you are doing or have been doing, i.e. an ***easing factor***. Continue to ask yourself the same question until you notice a pattern emerge. As soon as you start thinking something along the lines of:

"Oh, it seems to be whenever I do…my pain feels better"

encourage this particular activity or posture little and often throughout the day, as it is something your body likes and is therefore providing it with the ideal conditions to heal itself.

Just to summarise, ***you need to listen to your pain…***

➤ If it's at its normal level, you are not interested as this tells you nothing.

➤ If it is worse than normal, make a note of what you are/have been doing as this is an ***aggravating factor***.

➤ If it is better than normal, make a note of what you are/have been doing as this is an ***easing factor***.

As soon as you see a pattern begin to emerge, you should…

Avoid or modify the aggravating factors

and

encourage the easing factors.

Maybe you're saying to yourself right now that there are some things that are impossible for you to avoid. For example, it may be an activity you need to carry out for your work. I genuinely appreciate and understand this. In such circumstances, all I ask is for you to 'analyse' this particular posture or activity you are adopting and then try to modify it towards a posture/activity that you know your body finds more comfortable. In addition to this, also try to break any particular aggravating factors up into smaller, more manageable parts. The chapter, **Practical Advice:** ***The Influence of Regular Day-to-day Activities on Your Pain*** *will highlight some potential alternatives for you.*

As already discussed, by avoiding the aggravating postures and activities, you will be stopping yourself from interfering with the healing process. Also, by encouraging the easing factors you will be setting up the ideal conditions for your body to heal itself. Ultimately it is down to you; if you feel you cannot avoid or modify certain activities that aggravate your pain, you need to prioritise your pain against those aggravating activities.

Sorry to use another cliché but:

If you keep on doing what you've always done, you'll keep on getting what you've always got.

I'm sure you'll understand what I am saying here. If you are reading this book because you are suffering with low back pain and/or sciatica (and maybe you have been for some time) I can state without any shadow of a doubt why you are suffering with this level of pain: it is because you are creating the ideal conditions for it to be maintained.

Therefore, if you want this level of pain to change for the better you need to change the things you are doing. Once again, I appreciate this can be difficult sometimes, but that's why you need to start prioritising your pain over your day-to-day activities. If you do, it will not be long before you begin to notice the benefits.

I would just like to add a couple of important things before you read on:

  i)   If your pain feels particularly better or worse and you look back to see what you are or have been doing, please do not say to yourself you have been doing nothing…you are never doing 'nothing' unless you vanish from the face of the earth! Although it frustrates me when patients say this, I do understand what they mean. Usually it means not doing much; a classic example of this is sitting in front of the TV. If this is the case, you are not 'doing nothing', you are sitting in front of the TV. If you do not know by now, you will do fairly soon, sitting can be one of the most stressful things for low back pain and sciatica.

       You will also find out as you continue to read this book that telling yourself you were sitting when your pain felt better/worse may not be enough. You may need to be specific about the chair you were sitting in (was it soft or firm, high or low?) or the position your feet were in (were they flat on the floor or up on a stool?) and so on. All will be explained in more than adequate detail as you continue to read through this book, and in particular in the course of the chapter, **Practical Advice:** *The Influence of Regular Day-to-day Activities on Your Pain*.

ii)   Do not simply tell yourself your low back/sciatica is always painful, although I do appreciate it may always be painful! With regard to aggravating and easing factors, we are talking about degrees of pain. Therefore, if you are always in pain, you need to ask yourself what you are or have been doing when your pain increases or decreases a little, as it is these changes which will help identify the aggravating and easing factors.

Something I often ask patients is:

"What would you instinctively do should your low back/ sciatica be particularly painful?"

As far as I am concerned, the body naturally does its utmost to free ourselves of pain. Therefore, quite often, if we feel an increased level of pain, our body will subconsciously tell us what to do.

A classic example of this would be how the individual who has been sitting for some time with their back curved into a soft chair would automatically lean backwards to 'stretch' themselves out after rising from that chair. This is the body's way of telling you your lower back has been flexed for too long and therefore needs to be extended a little.

In a nutshell, if you find that you tend to perform a certain activity, or maybe place yourself in a certain position in order to ease your pain, there is every chance it is this type of position or activity that is an easing factor: therefore encourage it. Do not wait for your pain to increase before adopting these positions or performing these activities; perform them even when your pain is not present or not so bad, as the likelihood is this will help keep the pain away.

Are you still finding it difficult to elicit any particular aggravating or easing factors?

Most importantly, do not give up, as there are very few people who do not have them. Without wanting to sound patronising, you really need to scrutinise and analyse everything you are and have been doing when you notice any increase or decrease in your pain. If you have exhausted these but are still struggling to find anything, some patients have found the following questions useful...

What would you do throughout the course of the day if you really wanted to stir up your pain?

Quite often I would hear things such as they would perform plenty of housework, walk around the shops for a few hours, cut the grass, etc. If you can give some answers to this question, there is your starting point for finding some aggravating factors.

A similar question applies if you are struggling to find any easing factors...

What would you do through the course of the day if you wanted your low back pain/sciatica to be as comfortable as possible?

Once again, if you know what you would do to answer this question, you have a starting point for some easing factors.

DO I NEED TO AVOID THESE AGGRAVATING ACTIVITIES FOREVER?

I am pleased to tell you the answer to this question is an unequivocal **NO**. The reason for this, once again, is down to the human body. Let me explain…

The more we take these aggravating factors away from the structures causing pain, the more healing there will be. The more healing taking place, the stronger these structures will become and therefore the less pain you will feel. If you are feeling less pain, this means those same structures are less sensitive and therefore not being aggravated as easily and if they are not being aggravated as much, once again more healing will take place.

You will now find that activities which used to aggravate your pain no longer do so, because healing has taken place and your back is stronger. Therefore, I am happy for you to perform these activities, being sensible of course, and avoiding any unnecessary poor postures and activities. This is because the more controlled stresses you place across the structures which were responsible for your pain, the stronger those same structures will become.

I often use the analogy here of a sports person, let's say a sprinter, who injures himself. If he has torn a Hamstring muscle, for example, during his rehabilitation does he just keep on running even though it is causing him pain? No, of course he doesn't. The reason he does not is because he knows if he were to do this his Hamstring is going to take a lot longer to heal because he is aggravating it… . Ring any bells? It should do by now.

Therefore, this individual would rest his Hamstring muscle. Would he just completely rest it for six weeks or so until it was pain-free and then immediately compete in the next available race? Once again, of course he wouldn't. We all know if he were to do this the chances are his Hamstring wouldn't last very long until it tore again. This is because although it had healed, it would have only healed relative to the stresses placed upon it, i.e. very little.

Without wanting to labour the point, this individual would rest his Hamstring by avoiding any aggravating activities **BUT** as it healed he would place more and more appropriate stresses across it, e.g. walking, light jogging, running etc. until he was up to scratch and sprinting before the next race. The reason is that the body heals itself according to the stresses placed upon it; therefore, by slowly placing increased stresses upon it as it heals, it will heal much more strongly.

My point here is that this is exactly what I want you to do with your lower back/sciatic nerve. As your body heals itself and becomes stronger, activities that were aggravating factors will no longer be so. Therefore, as long as you're sensible, I want you to carry out as many of your normal day-to-day activities as you can… *as long as they do not aggravate your pain.*

We will now be achieving a positive cycle of the pain healing itself which leads to the structures involved becoming stronger. With these structures being stronger it means there are fewer aggravating factors and because there are fewer aggravating factors the body will be able to continue to heal itself and so on…

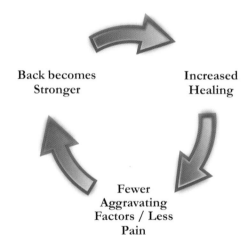

Back becomes
Stronger

Increased
Healing

Fewer
Aggravating
Factors / Less
Pain

This is opposite to the negative vicious cycle of increased inflammation and decreased healing shown on **page 60** of the chapter, **Learning Zone: *Why You are Feeling Pain***.

By carrying out the advice given throughout this chapter, you will be able to settle down your pain considerably.

The following chapter is **Step Four:** *How to Diagnose Your Pain*. This section of the book will empower you with the knowledge to provide yourself with a functional diagnosis for your low back pain and/or sciatica. This specific diagnosis you give yourself will be the foundation upon which you base your subsequent exercise programme. This chapter will also explain the concepts of FDP and EDP mentioned in previous chapters.

Step Four:

How to Diagnose Your Pain

Okay, so from the previous chapters you will now be aware that your body's own healing process is without doubt the greatest healer known to man. As long as you give yourself the correct conditions, your body will begin to heal itself. What you need to do now is provide yourself with a functional diagnosis so you are more specifically aware of why you are suffering with pain.

This in turn will enable you to care for your body twenty-four hours a day, by placing the appropriate postural stresses upon it and prescribing yourself specific exercises to ensure your back becomes stronger and more supple. This will not only help resolve your pain, but also help to eliminate the chances of it recurring again.

The body really is fantastic, it does everything for us. As long as you listen to your body, it will more or less spell out the diagnosis for you.

Having had many years of experience studying and treating individuals with low back pain and sciatica, I can confidently say from a functional point of view they can nearly all be grouped together within two diagnostic categories:

Flexion Dominated Pain (FDP)

and

Extension Dominated Pain (EDP)

These two diagnoses are differentiated by the typical movement patterns which tend to aggravate the pain. A description can be seen in **Appendix II: *Glossary of Terms***; however, in a nutshell, *flexion* refers to the process of bending forward and *extension* refers to the process of leaning backwards. These are the two principle movements which tend to cause most low back pain and sciatica.

By principle movements, I mean it is not only purely bending forward or leaning backwards that causes the pain, but rather any movement or posture that has a similar influence upon your lower back.

I have listed below some typical functional activities that can be grouped under the diagnoses of FDP or EDP. However, more examples can be found in the following chapter, **Practical Advice:** *The Influence of Regular Day-to-day Activities on Your Pain*.

Flexion Dominated Pain

Bending/Leaning forward
Sitting for long periods, especially in soft or low chairs
Vacuuming
Making the bed /Cleaning the bath
Driving, especially for long periods

Extension Dominated Pain

Leaning backwards
Lying on your stomach, especially if resting up on your elbows
Walking, especially downhill or in high heels
Reaching up
Swimming breaststroke

It is important to mention that these activities are not set in stone. They are just a guide to some typical aggravating postures and activities for the given functional diagnosis.

I could probably add a third diagnostic category here, namely, **Rotational Dominated Pain (RDP)**. This is where the lower back lacks stability, not just in the planes of moving forwards or backwards, but more so in combined movements, typically rotation to either side.

Although I have encountered RDP a few times when treating patients, I have rarely found it to be the primary cause of someone's pain.

The situation usually arises when the patient is suffering predominately with FDP or EDP and there is an underlying element of RDP. As you progress through this book and work on the appropriate exercises, in particular those given in **Step Seven:** *Moving Forward with Core Stability Exercises*, your back will develop the strength and suppleness which will address any RDP element present, as well as the primary FDP or EDP.

You may now be raising your eyebrows a little and thinking: *'No way, there are far more than two or three things that can go wrong with my back.'* If you are thinking this, I couldn't agree with you more.

However, I need to emphasise the point that these are *functional diagnoses* I am giving here, not specific medical ones. I could go further and give a more specific diagnosis, such as those given in **Appendix I:** *Glossary of Diagnostic Terms* but it really isn't relevant, as it would make no difference to how you treat your pain.

If I can just pose myself two questions:

1. Has every patient I have treated with FDP or EDP had the same medical diagnosis?

2. Have the fundamental principles of their treatment been the same?

I can answer them both unequivocally.

The answer to the first question is undoubtedly no. There are many different medical diagnoses I have encountered while treating the many patients I have. However, it is important I hastily answer the second question with a yes, as the fundamental principles are the same no matter what the medical diagnosis is. That is, providing the body with the optimum conditions in which it can heal itself and then prescribing an appropriate exercise programme that will further reduce inappropriate stresses and address the cause of the problem. This approach will lead not only to the pain resolving itself, but, of equal importance, the elimination of risk factors which result in recurring problems.

My point being here is that you do not need to be given a specific medical diagnosis to be able to resolve your low back pain or sciatica. Besides, whenever you see any therapist or consultant, the diagnosis you are given is only a hypothesis…

Even if you have had an MRI scan and it shows you are suffering with a prolapsed disc, it still doesn't necessarily mean this is the cause of your pain! I know you may find this hard to believe, but it is widely accepted within the health profession that there are many people walking around who are suffering with prolapsed discs and yet are feeling no pain at all.

Also, why is it that two different people can be suffering with low back pain and be diagnosed with a prolapsed disc following an MRI scan, yet after they have both had the prolapsed disc removed, one may still be suffering in pain and yet the other may be pain-free? The answer to this is that for the former person the disc bulge was not actually the cause of the pain, even though it was quite apparent a prolapsed disc was present.

DO I NEED AN EXACT MEDICAL DIAGNOSIS TO BEGIN USING THIS BOOK?

Not necessarily: as I have just mentioned, whenever any health professional provides you with a given diagnosis, it is still only a hypothesis. I really want to reinforce that everything you are reading within this book is exactly how I would carry out an assessment and subsequent treatment, just as if we were standing face-to-face in a physiotherapy department. The detail I go into here is exactly the same. The only difference is that by reading this book, you do not have the opportunity to ask me further questions with regard to any more information you may require.

Is this a disadvantage? With regard to resolving your pain I would say an unequivocal no. With regard to resolving your curiosity for specific knowledge, which I can understand, then the answer could be yes. I say 'could be' as it is important for me to stress that although I am not there with you to answer any specific questions, I have made every conceivable effort to ensure that all the information you need know to free yourself of pain is within this book. I would also add I have provided more information than most patients ever request anyway.

Okay, you should now be comfortable with the fact it is more than adequate to choose between one of two functional diagnoses for the pain you are suffering, those diagnoses being FDP and EDP. The remainder of this chapter will show you how to self-diagnose your back problem, and therefore decide whether your pain is FDP or EDP related.

PROVIDING YOURSELF WITH A FUNCTIONAL DIAGNOSIS

The first thing I need you to do is to think about the activities/postures that you feel most aggravate your pain, in order to establish which category your pain falls into. As I have previously mentioned, typical examples of these can be found in the following chapter, **Practical Advice:** *The Influence of Regular Day-to-day Activities on Your Pain*. However, it is important to work them out for yourself also, as ultimately it is the position of *your spine* while performing these activities that will dictate whether you are suffering from FDP or EDP.

The reason I say this is that even though, for example an activity may be typically flexion-related, the way you carry that activity out may be with an over-extended spine. Consequently, if you were to take it for granted that such an activity was related to FDP, yet you were carrying it out with an extended spine, you would probably be misdiagnosing your pain.

Once again I will refer you to the following chapter, **Practical Advice:** *The Influence of Regular Day-to-day Activities on Your Pain* as this chapter will describe specific activities and how they may vary with regard to FDP or EDP. The most important thing though is to listen to your body and try to 'feel' what your back is doing. You will become more adept at doing this as you read through this book and have a further understanding as to how your back moves and the influences tight and weak muscles have upon it.

The previous chapter **Step Three:** *How to Optimise Your Body's Healing Potential* explained how best to work out what your aggravating and easing factors are. By analysing these and thinking about whether your back tends to be more flexed or more extended during the given activities or postures, it will help guide you towards your specific diagnosis.

What if I cannot work out what aggravates my pain…?

If you have analysed things to the best of your ability and yet you are still unable to work out what type of activity it is that causes you to have increased pain, you may need to try a few different things while your pain is particularly bad.

You will have read earlier in this chapter **(page 102)** five examples of typical activities which may cause pain in someone suffering with either FDP or EDP. If you are finding it difficult to elicit which activities may be responsible for aggravating your pain in the first place, wait until your pain is particularly bad and then carry out some of those given activities. If, as you do so, you notice one or two of them tend to increase or decrease your pain a little, use that information with regard to providing yourself with a functional diagnosis.

If a certain activity tends to make your pain worse, it is likely that the movement related to that activity is your specific diagnosis, e.g. if extension-related activities aggravate your pain, it is likely you are suffering with EDP. On the other hand, if a particular activity eases your pain, it is more likely to be the opposite of the diagnosis you are suffering with, e.g. if extension-related activities ease your pain, it is likely you are suffering with FDP.

As a clinical example, I was treating a patient who only suffered low back pain at night; she had looked at all the things she was doing before going to bed, etc. and was unable to say whether her pain was FDP or EDP related. On asking her what she definitely would or would not do when the pain woke her at night, almost instantly she told me she would definitely not lie on her stomach, as this would make things worse. That immediately made me think that it could well be EDP she was suffering from, due to prone lying encouraging extension of the back. (See the chapter, **Practical Advice:** *Do Not Replace Your Bed*.)

To reinforce this, she then commented that she would sit herself on the edge of her bed with her elbows resting on her knees if her pain became too unbearable, in order to ease the pain a little. This is a typically flexion-related position that tends to ease those suffering with EDP, further reinforcing my initial thoughts. We then went on to look for any particular muscle imbalances and encouraged the principles and exercises appropriate for someone with EDP…her pain resolved itself very quickly.

WHAT IF YOU GET THIS DIAGNOSIS WRONG?

It's no problem. If you misdiagnose your pain and therefore prescribe yourself with the incorrect exercises, it really is nothing to worry about. Okay, I'm not going to say it isn't going to make your pain a little sore. In fact, I can almost guarantee that if you perform the incorrect exercises, it will increase your pain a little. However, as long as you ease yourself into the exercises, as I always recommend you do, it will soon settle down again.

Remember also, one of the main principles of this book is that the 'No-Pain, No-Gain' approach is a myth (see the final chapter, **Old Wives' Tales**). Therefore, as soon as you feel any particular activities or exercises are aggravating your signs and symptoms, it is important to ease off.

I'm sure there have been many times when you have done the wrong thing for your low back pain/sciatica and therefore aggravated your pain… did it settle down again afterwards? I would say it definitely did. This time will be no different, and as long as you ease yourself into the exercises, it should again settle down pretty quickly.

I hope this doesn't sound too flippant, but to take a positive from this I would say you are now a step closer to resolving your pain! This is because you have just established some aggravating factors for your pain and therefore know what type of exercises not to do. Not just that but let's say, for example, the exercises were ones for someone suffering with FDP, i.e. extension-based exercises, and yet they aggravated your pain, there are only two possible scenarios:

i)   You are suffering with FDP, it is just that you performed the appropriate exercises too aggressively or too soon. If this is the case, wait for your pain to settle and then re-introduce a gentler exercise for FDP or perform the same exercise but ease off a little.

ii)   You are not suffering with FDP. If this is the case, once again wait for your pain to settle down and then gently introduce the appropriate exercises for someone suffering with EDP.

Point i) will be covered again in the chapter, **Learning Zone: *The Principles of Exercise*** but it is important for me to point out from the start that if any postures, exercises or activities do aggravate your pain, they may still be the correct ones to perform. The reason they may have aggravated your pain could simply be because you tried a few too many or attempted them too soon. Under these circumstances, you need to perform the same exercises again when your pain has settled down, but ease off on them a little.

Another example to highlight this point, only using EDP this time, is bending forward. With regard to EDP, it is often the case that the soft tissues in the lower back itself and associated structures are tight and need stretching out. Therefore, an exercise such as a forward flexion in sitting (**page 197 in Step Five: *Getting Moving Again***) may well be given. However, if you were to perform too many of these, your pain may increase due to you stretching these structures too much too soon. This does not mean you have now developed FDP, rather you still have EDP but you performed this particular exercise too soon or have performed too many of them.

Aggravating and easing factors are also very specific to how you perform the given activity. For example, if you were to walk for 5-10 minutes and this eased your pain, then walking for 5-10 minutes is an easing factor. If you were then to walk for 15-20 minutes and this began to aggravate your pain, then walking for 15-20 minutes is an aggravating factor. My point here is that it is not walking that is an easing or aggravating factor, but rather how long you walk for.

When you feel you have a good idea as to your functional diagnosis, think to yourself how you would feel if you were to perform any of the following activities:

i)   Bending forwards (sitting or standing)
ii) Hugging your knees to your chest
iii) Lying on your stomach
iv) Gently leaning backwards

If your 'gut instinct' is that i) and ii) would definitely aggravate your pain, there is a very good chance you are suffering with FDP.

If your 'gut instinct' is that iii) and iv) would definitely aggravate your pain, there is a very good chance you are suffering with EDP.

In addition to this, there is a fair chance that if both i) and ii) aggravate your pain, then iii) and iv) may ease your pain and vice versa. I will elaborate on this further a little later in this chapter.

As always, I have to say this is not set in stone, therefore get a good feel about how your pain responds to more than just the examples given above. Nevertheless, these examples are classic activities associated with FDP and EDP.

> *With regard to EDP, I often hear patients complain of their back feeling 'weak' or that there is a kind of 'constant ache' in their lower back. Once again this is only a rule of thumb, but if you recognise these signs and symptoms, you may well be suffering with EDP.*

The really important thing I wish to stress here is 'gut instinct', i.e. listen to what your body is telling you. As I have mentioned before, we are all unique individuals. It would make my job so much easier as a physiotherapist, if we were all created from a production line like motor vehicles and were therefore identical. As soon as someone turned up with such and such a pain we could then type it into a computer or turn to Page X of the 'Human Body Manual' and we would know exactly what to do. Unfortunately, the human body is not like this and that is why we are so special. The best person to know what is wrong with them is *you*, as you are the only one who can feel what is going on.

On the subject of listening to your body and being guided by what it tells you, we sometimes instinctively do what is best for us without even knowing it. Bearing this in mind, if your pain is particularly bad and the natural thing for you to do is to lean backwards or maybe lie on your stomach, there is a fair chance you are suffering with FDP. This is because leaning backwards and lying on your stomach are typically extension-based postures. We will be using extension-based exercises to treat FDP. Therefore, if your natural instinct is to extend your lower back to ease your pain, the likelihood is you are suffering with FDP.

Alternatively, if, when your pain is particularly bad, the instinctive thing for you to do is sit down and rest forward on your knees or maybe lie down and hug your knees up to your chest, there is a fair chance you are suffering with EDP. This is because of principles similar to the ones outlined above. Sitting forward on a chair or hugging your knees to your chest are flexion-based postures. If it is postures/exercises such as these which ease your pain, the likelihood is that you are suffering with EDP, as we will be using flexion-based postures and exercises to treat EDP.

CONFIRMING YOUR DIAGNOSIS

To confirm further your diagnosis, I would like you to try the following simple exercises in relation to the diagnosis you feel you are suffering with. As you perform each exercise, I want you to best describe the sensation you are feeling, be it in your back, buttock or down your leg.

The following examples may not be very useful if you are suffering from acute inflammatory pain, where everything seems to hurt. If you are, it is probably best to return to **Step 2: *How to STOP Acutely Inflamed Pain*** *in order to settle your pain down. As soon as it starts to settle and you feel you need to confirm your diagnosis, return to this chapter.*

Flexion Dominated Pain

PRONE LYING

The first position I would suggest you try would be lying on your front with a pillow or two underneath your stomach. This will encourage extension of your lower back, but the pillow(s) will prevent your back from over extending.

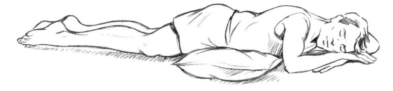

If you find this makes little or no difference, then try removing one or both pillows to see if that is easier; maybe so you are lying on your stomach as shown below. As always we are looking for a reduction of your signs and symptoms.

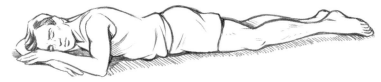

If you feel that there is still very little improvement (but things are not getting worse) try propping yourself up a little higher, maybe with a pillow under your forearms or resting on your elbows (as shown below). Either way, once again we would be looking for a decrease in your pain if you are suffering with FDP.

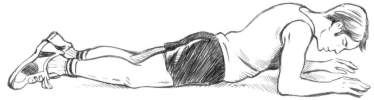

Extension Dominated Pain

SITTING FORWARDS RESTING ON YOUR KNEES

If this position relieves your pain or you feel a stretching/pulling sensation around your lower back, buttock or upper-leg area, there is a fair chance your diagnosis is correct and you are suffering with EDP. If there is no change to your pain, try leaning further forwards, maybe try to touch the floor with your fingers or even pass your hands underneath the chair and behind you. Once again, I would be looking for a decrease in your pain or a stretching sensation around your back, buttock or leg area.

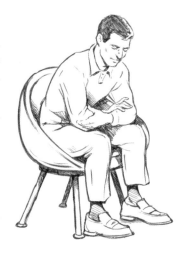

An alternative position is to lie on your back and hug one knee to your chest.

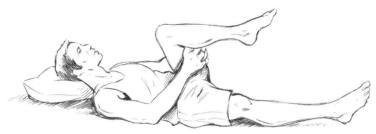

You could also hug both knees together up to your chest.

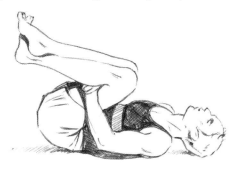

Once again, you should be looking for a reduction in your pain or a stretching/pulling sensation around your lower back, buttock or upper leg area. If so, there is a fair chance your diagnosis is correct and you are suffering with EDP.

NB. If there is no reduction in pain, rather just a stretching sensation you feel, be careful as this is not a guarantee you are suffering with EDP. In some circumstances FDP can give feelings of stretching around the lower back region. In such cases where you are still a little unsure, I would simply ask you to *gently* repeat this bending forward/knees to chest movement about 5 or 6 times. If, as you do this, you feel you can gradually move further and/or the pain and stretching decreases, the chances are you are suffering with EDP.

If, on the other hand, your pain increases as you perform these movements, the chances are it is either FDP you are suffering with, or your back is still relatively inflamed. Therefore, I would ask you to either try the previous exercises for FDP and see whether they ease your pain at all, or return to **Step Two:** *How to STOP Acutely Inflamed Pain* in order to settle further your discomfort.

These are very good indicators for FDP and EDP, and, if your symptoms do ease when you perform the relevant position/exercise for your diagnosis, there is a very good chance you are correct and are suffering with that diagnosis. Therefore, continue to read this book with that diagnosis in mind.

Equally, if either of the previous examples aggravate your pain (and there is a fair chance one set will tend to ease your pain and the other will aggravate it) it is likely that that movement is giving you your diagnosis. For example, the positions given for easing EDP are *flexion–dominated* positions. If any of these aggravate your pain, the chances are it is FDP you are suffering with and not EDP. The opposite is obviously true, in that we use *extension-dominated* positions to ease FDP. Therefore, if these extension-dominated positions aggravate your pain, it is likely you are suffering from EDP and not FDP.

The main reasons for providing yourself with the appropriate diagnosis are twofold:

i) **To enable you to know which type of activities to encourage or avoid.**

As I have mentioned before, those activities that aggravate FDP are likely to ease EDP and vice versa. Therefore, I would like you to avoid those activities that aggravate your pain and encourage those that ease your pain, i.e. if you are suffering with FDP, as a rule of thumb you need to avoid flexion-dominated positions and encourage extension-dominated positions, whereas if you are suffering with EDP, you need to avoid extension-dominated positions and encourage flexion-dominated positions. (See the following chapter, **Practical Advice:** *The Influence of Regular Day-to-day Activities on Your Pain* for an outline of what typical day-to-day activities tend to be more flexion or extension based.)

ii) **To ensure you prescribe yourself with the correct exercises.**

These exercises are provided throughout this book, beginning with **Step Five:** *Getting Moving Again*.

Before we move on to the following chapter, **Practical Advice:** *The Influence of Regular Day-to-day Activities on Your Pain* I wish to finish this chapter with an explanation of the two diagnoses used throughout this book. This will allow you to understand why you are experiencing your pain and how, by using the advice and exercises provided by this book, you will be able to resolve your pain as well.

DIAGNOSTIC DEFINITIONS

If you are able to understand why you are suffering pain, along with what is happening to your body while you are carrying out your self-prescribed exercise programme, this will help with your understanding of how to alleviate your pain.

When treating people within the physiotherapy department, I always make sure I give as thorough an explanation as I can to enable the patient to really understand why they are experiencing pain and why I am asking them to perform certain exercises/activities in order to reduce their pain.

As soon as they understand this, it is half the battle, as they will now know why they are doing the exercises as opposed to performing them simply because I ask them to. Not only does this increase understanding, it also increases compliance of the advice/exercises which are given.

This is exactly why I wish to finish this chapter with an explanation of FDP and EDP. I will give the best examples of how to understand each of these causes of pain and why I provide the given exercises for each individual diagnosis.

> *It is important for me to state here that, as I mentioned previously, there are many medical reasons as to why you may be in pain. As you will know, I feel these different medical reasons or diagnoses can be banded into the two functional diagnoses of FDP and EDP. For my explanation as to what is happening, I am going to use what I believe are the two most common 'medical' causes of FDP and EDP.*

Flexion Dominated Pain

I use the herniated disc medical diagnosis to explain this one, as I feel it is probably the main cause of this type of pain and it also explains wonderfully the principles of how the treatment works. FDP problems are usually a result of too much flexion, typically bending forward and sitting.

This increased pressure on the back tends to squeeze or pinch together the anterior aspect of the two vertebra above and below the disc, yet 'open up' the posterior aspect of the same vertebra. This in turn has a squeezing-like effect on the disc between these vertebra, which encourages the disc itself to bulge from its normal position, as shown below.

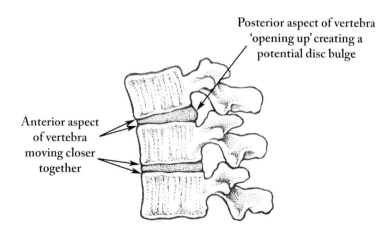

Posterior aspect of vertebra 'opening up' creating a potential disc bulge

Anterior aspect of vertebra moving closer together

I sometimes describe this as being similar to how an inner tube may bulge out from a weak spot in a tyre. As soon as the disc begins to bulge, it can become inflamed, therefore creating pain in the lower back. If this bulging of the disc and subsequent inflammation begins to encroach upon the adjacent nerves that pass down the leg, then pain, pins and needles and/or numbness can also be felt anywhere along the distribution of that particular nerve.

This is where the term sciatica comes from, i.e. pain along the distribution of the sciatic nerve. As described in **Step Two:** *How to STOP Acutely Inflamed Pain* the first aim of treatment is simply to decrease the inflammation in order to decrease the pain and sensitivity present.

As the inflammation and therefore sensitivity decreases, we then need to work on reducing the bulging disc back to its natural position, i.e. solely between the adjacent vertebral bodies and not protruding at all outside of them. This is why, for this type of diagnosis, we use an extension-based exercise programme.

Let's go back a little with regard to the cause of this herniated disc. I will ask you to place your hands horizontally in front of you with the palms facing each other about two to three inches apart and your fingers pointing away from you.

Now imagine each hand represents a lumbar vertebra, with your fingers being the front of the vertebra and the heel of your hands being the back of the vertebra. The space between your hands is where the disc would sit.

Every time we bend forward or sit in a poorly flexed posture, the spine bends in a manner that is the equivalent of tilting your fingertips towards each other and pulling the heel of your hands apart.

As you do this, I am sure you can imagine how this 'squeezing' effect on the front (fingertips) of the two adjacent vertebra would encourage the disc to bulge backwards (towards the heel of your hands). It is this bulging that results in increased stress upon the disc and tissues about the posterior aspect of the back, which can then lead to inflammation and subsequent pain.

The most important thing we need to do now is reduce the bulging disc back to its natural position between the vertebra. This is why the exercise programme is extension based. If we can reverse that pinching effect, by extending the lumbar spine instead of flexing it, this will encourage the disc to return to its correct position.

By doing this it will be the equivalent of placing the heel of your hands closer together and your fingertips further apart, therefore helping to squeeze the disc back into its correct position.

Unfortunately, it is not always quite as simple as this as the structures involved may be extremely inflamed and therefore sensitive. This, along with the fact there may be a particularly large disc bulge present, means the extension exercises themselves may 'pinch' the disc too much, too soon, and therefore aggravate the signs and symptoms.

A classic example to highlight this would be if you were suffering with FDP and were to sit in a soft low chair for a considerable time. As you were in this position, you would be encouraging the disc to bulge backwards in the manner just described. If you were then to stand up, the posterior aspect of the adjacent vertebra would begin to close together (heel of the hands) just as the treatment principle encourages.

However, if they close together too much too soon, particularly if there is a sizeable disc bulge or if the disc is very inflamed and sensitive, the disc will not like this squeezing action as it becomes pinched and therefore there will be an increased amount of pain.

With this sitting to standing example, the individual will typically find it difficult to stand up straight immediately and will assume a flexed or 'crouched over' type posture. Yet after several steps they will slowly but surely begin to straighten up. This is because the initial standing up pinched the disc too much, hence the increased pain. However, as the disc is gradually 'squeezed' back into a better position, the pain – and therefore the ability to stand up correctly – eases.

This pattern of movement, where standing from sitting can be initially painful but then ease off as we begin to move, can also be present for those suffering with EDP. (I have warned you nothing is straightforward with the human body!) This highlights the need to be aware of how your back responds to many different activities and not just one. Nevertheless, although the signs and symptoms are similar, the reasons for them are completely different, and I will explain this later in the chapter.

This example of the disc being pinched too much, too soon is also the reason why I ask you to place a pillow under your stomach if prone lying is too painful, as given in the earlier treatment example for FDP.

This is because sometimes, during the early stages of treatment, prone lying can cause the vertebrae to pinch on the disc too much, too soon. By placing the pillow under your stomach, however, it helps reduce the downward arching effect on your back. This in turn helps to decrease the pinching effect.

This is the main principle upon which the treatment of FDP is based. It is a progressive set of extension exercises which gradually ease the disc into its natural position, thereby decreasing the stress upon those structures involved and allowing healing to take place.

As the healing takes place, the vulnerable areas of the disc that allowed the bulge to occur will strengthen. Consequently, at a later date when similar stresses may be placed upon the disc, due to its now renewed strength, the disc will be able to tolerate these stresses and therefore no bulge will occur and no pain will be felt.

I am sure you can now imagine how, if you were to continue with increased flexion activities, it would further encourage the disc to bulge and therefore lead to increased pain and sensitivity, and possibly further referred pain down the leg. The weakened areas of the disc would also be given no opportunity to heal themselves.

Extension-Dominated Pain

For this functional diagnosis, I use facet joint pain as the medical example: once again because it is probably the most common cause of EDP and also because it highlights well the principles of treatment given for EDP throughout this book.

EDP is usually a result of too much extension of the lumbar spine. This is typically a result of poor posture, for example having an increased lumbar lordosis when standing, and weak core stability muscles. If the core stability muscles are weak, the pelvis tends to rotate forwards, which is in effect extension of the lower back. For further explanations on this see the chapter, **Learning Zone: *Why Muscles are the Key Factor in Eliminating Your Pain*.**

When the back is in the extended position, it forces the surfaces of the adjacent facet joints against one another, as shown below.

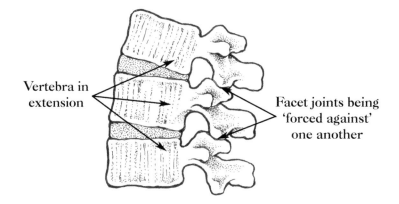

Vertebra in extension

Facet joints being 'forced against' one another

To enable you to visualise this cause of EDP, I am going to ask you to place your hands two to three inches apart as you did when you visualised FDP (with the heel of your hands being the posterior aspect of the vertebra and your fingers the anterior part).

This time, however, I am going to ask you to move the heel of your hands towards each other. This is similar to what happens to adjacent vertebrae when the lumbar spine is in the extended position, which then forces the facet joints against one another and can ultimately lead to pain.

Although the body is designed to tolerate these stresses, just as the discs are with repeated flexion, if these stresses are repeated too often, they will breach the body's pain threshold level and therefore pain will result.

When pain does occur, there is every chance that significant inflammation will also be present; subsequent increased sensitivity and muscle tightness about the lower back and facet joints may then follow. These tight muscles place yet more increased stresses upon the facet joints, which aggravate the structures further; this then leads to more pain and inflammation and so on.

Using a similar principle to that given earlier for FDP, the aim is to reverse these stresses present, only this time we will reverse them by flexing the lumbar spine in order to separate the facet joints. This will be the equivalent of pointing the tips of your fingers towards each other and placing the heel of your hands further apart. As we separate the facet joints, there will be less stress upon them and therefore less pain and more chance of healing taking place.

Not only this, but as healing takes place and the sensitivity decreases, we will then need to increase the flexion further in order to stretch out any tight soft tissues which may be present. When these tight soft tissues are stretched, they will no longer place increased stresses upon the facet joints, therefore the likelihood of further healing taking place is once again increased. As well as stretching the appropriate structures, it is important that core stability exercises are also performed as part of the rehabilitation.

I am sure you can now imagine how, if you were to continue adopting extension-related movements and postures, it would continue to place inappropriate stresses upon the facet joints and therefore little healing would take place and your pain would increase.

*One particular medical diagnosis that I would class under EDP is Lumbar Spinal Stenosis (See **Appendix I: Glossary of Diagnostic Terms**). This is a condition which is aggravated intensely by walking and eased almost immediately by sitting or leaning forward. If you feel you may be suffering with this you need to speak to your GP, as this condition does not always respond well to the exercises given in this book. You would definitely gain some relief by encouraging flexion-based postures and exercises, but this relief may only be temporary and no long-term benefit may be gained.*

In summary, if you are suffering with FDP you need to encourage extension, whereas if you are suffering with EDP you need to encourage flexion. However, as I have mentioned previously, nothing is straightforward with the human body, and you can have too much of a good thing.

As I explained with FDP, if you try to extend your back too much, too soon, or for too long, you may begin to aggravate your pain. The same is true when we use flexion to treat EDP, especially if the main source of your pain is a result of tight muscles placing increased stresses upon the facet joints.

For this latter example, I often use the analogy of bending your finger back. If you were to bend one of your fingers back, the likelihood is you will not feel pain but rather a stretching sensation across the joints. If, however, you were to keep that finger bent back for say a minute or more, the likelihood is you would begin to feel pain across those same joints.

This brings me back to the example I mentioned on **page 118** with regard to FDP, whereby prolonged sitting can lead to pain and difficulty in standing up afterwards due to the increased 'pinching' on the disc as you stand up.

If you are suffering with EDP and have tight muscles in your lower back, when you initially sit down you may actually feel some relief as the facet joints are slightly 'pulled apart'. However, if you were to sit in this position for too long, it will have the same effect as bending your finger back for too long, i.e. you may begin to experience pain. As you then stand up you may once again, just as with FDP, find it initially difficult and painful to do so.

I will refer again to the example of bending a finger back. If I were to do this quite firmly for a good few minutes, the chances are not only would I feel pain but also if I were to try and make a fist immediately afterwards, it would be painful and difficult to clench the finger which I was bending back. After a few attempts, however, it would gradually bend okay and I would be able to make a fist with no problems (please do not try this to the detriment of your finger, I have used this as an example for you to simply relate to!).

Something very similar can happen if you are suffering with EDP and stand up after prolonged sitting. Initially you would find it difficult and painful to do so, yet after a few steps you would find it easier until eventually you could stand up okay. This is a result of you over-stretching the structures concerned.

The main difference between FDP & EDP with regard to prolonged sitting, is that with FDP if you were to sit on a soft low chair, it would not take long at all for your pain to increase. However, if you were suffering with EDP the likelihood is that initially you would find it quite a comfortable position, even though it may feel a little tight across your lower back. Only after a significant period of time would your pain levels begin to increase.

NB. It is also important for me to mention that the body is designed to be able to both flex and extend the lumbar spine as we go about our day

-to-day activities. However, it is only when one of these movements is 'abused' whereby it is either performed too many times within a short period or maybe fewer times but for very prolonged periods that pain results. The reason for me highlighting this is because I do not want you to think you are in danger of curing one type of pain but then developing the opposite as you progress through the treatment exercises. For example, I do not want you to think that as you proceed with extension-based exercises for FDP, you are in danger of developing EDP due to the continued extension of the lumbar spine...

> ### *The key to all exercises given in this book is 'little and often' ...and the body, as I have mentioned, is more than capable of tolerating this.*

The first thing we need to do, whatever your diagnosis, is settle down any inflammation which is present. If we can do this, it will result in decreased pain and sensitivity of the structures involved. This will in turn enable you to progress further with the exercises provided in this book.

The following chapter, **Practical Advice:** *The Influence of Regular Day-to-day Activities on Your Pain,* will help facilitate the speed at which your body heals your pain. It will do so by covering the many typical day-to-day activities there are, and explain them with reference to both EDP and FDP. Consequently, this will help you with regard to recognising specific aggravating activities and determining whether they are typically flexion- or extension-based.

Practical Advice:

The Influence of Regular Day-to-day Activities on Your Pain

This chapter complements several others given throughout this book and in particular **Step Three:** *How to Optimise Your Body's Healing Potential*. This is because it gives you some typical day-to-day activities which can aggravate any low back pain or sciatica and explains whether they tend to be more flexion or extension dominated.

As I have mentioned many times before, the most important thing is for you to listen to and take note of what your body is telling you. This is because although the following is a very good guide as to whether the given activity is typically flexion or extension-based, ultimately it is *your* low back and/or sciatic nerve that is giving you pain and no one knows your body as well as you do. Therefore 'get a feel' for what position your back is in when carrying out the following activities and postures.

SITTING

I have put this 'activity' first because it is probably the most common aggravating position for someone suffering with low back pain or sciatica, yet it is something a lot of people tend to do when they are in pain, as they feel it is a good way to rest their back. The irony is that sitting can be one of the most stressful things you can do for low back pain or sciatica.

One particular patient I treated highlights this point well. He was a painter and decorator, and when he visited me for the first time he had already seen his pain ease, without treatment, to about the 75 per cent level, i.e. 75 per cent better. However, over the previous few months he was struggling to shake off this last 25 per cent and was becoming increasingly frustrated by it.

Following the assessment it became apparent he was suffering with FDP, yet he was not convinced by this diagnosis and my explanation. The reason for this was that he spent much of his day bending and could go some days at work with no problems at all and others with only 'little niggles' here and there.

I explained that, amongst other indicators, one of the reasons for me giving this diagnosis was that he said if he sat in his easy chair at home for any more than an hour (in a very flexed posture), his pain became 'unbearable' and he then had to get up and walk around. It was no surprise to me that when he did get up and walk around, his pain went away almost immediately.

Therefore, this individual could spend all of his working day bending, which would give him relatively few problems, yet he would then spend an hour or so in a chair and develop quite intense pain. This meant that sitting for an hour was more stressful for his back than his day at work painting and decorating!

The reason for this was that although he was bending a lot at work, he had to stand up quite often for one reason or another, therefore straightening himself up (standing is naturally an upright posture). By straightening himself up little and often throughout his day, he was continually taking stress away from his back, which is the likely reason as to why he felt little or no pain while at work. When he was at home, however, he was spending a prolonged period of time with his back in a flexed position sitting in his easy chair.

That was until his pain became unbearable, when he then decided to stand and straighten himself up, and guess what? When he did this his pain went away. The problem was he had not connected the two and therefore could not work out why his pain was better during the day when he was working and yet worse during the evening when he was doing 'nothing'.

I highlighted this to the patient, provided him with appropriate postural advice, which I will discuss shortly, along with a few simple stretches for him to perform (which are all given in **Step Six: *Move Forward with Stretching Exercises***) and within a few weeks the last 25 per cent of his pain, which he had been tolerating for several months, resolved itself.

The point of this example is you should never underestimate the stresses that sitting can have upon low back pain and sciatica. Many times while treating patients, I have found that a few simple corrections of posture, along with advice regarding eliminating prolonged postures, is enough to resolve their pain.

Fidgeting

*I have also had many patients tell me that sitting does not aggravate their pain, yet on further questioning it is quite apparent it does. The reason they have said it does not is because they say if they 'fidget around' it eases or takes the pain away. The fact they need to fidget tells me that sitting does aggravate their pain so…**do not fidget**! If you feel the need to fidget, your body is fed up with being sat down, therefore get yourself up and walk around a little.*

Before we continue any further, I feel I have to say it is usually the case that sitting tends to aggravate FDP. However, I'm afraid I am going to complicate things a little now, as it can also aggravate EDP. The reason for this is because if you are suffering with EDP as a result of tight muscles/ soft tissue across your lower back, when you sit down and place a flexion stress across your back it will begin to stretch these structures.

I often use the analogy here of bending one of your fingers back. If you were to do this it is unlikely to hurt, although you will probably feel some kind of stretching sensation across the joints. However, if you were to hold it there for a considerable length of time, the chances are it will become painful.

Exactly the same type of thing would happen if you were to sit for a long time while suffering with EDP as a result of tight muscles/soft tissue across your lower back. This is because just as the soft tissues in your finger can become over-stretched and painful, so can the tight soft tissues in your back. This, along with explanations of FDP and EDP, was explained in more detail during the previous chapter, **Step Four:** *How to Diagnose Your Pain*.

So how do you know whether you are suffering with FDP or EDP if sitting aggravates your pain?

Well first, as I have said before, no one particular posture or movement will give you a certain diagnosis. You need to take into account as many of the aggravating and easing factors as you can that best fit a certain diagnosis. However, there is a reasonable 'rule of thumb' you can use with regard to sitting and that is as follows:

If you are suffering with FDP and deliberately adopt a poor flexed posture, it will not take too long for your pain to increase. If, however, you are suffering with EDP and do the same thing, there is a fair chance that initially you will find it quite comfortable.

This is because if a disc bulge is responsible for your FDP, the increased flexed posture would exacerbate this bulge further, therefore increasing your pain. With EDP however, it is likely that compression of the facet joints is the cause of your pain. When you sit in a flexed posture, you will be 'pulling apart' the surfaces of the facet joints, therefore taking pressure from them and consequently reducing your pain (this was all explained in the previous chapter, **Step Four:** *How to Diagnose Your Pain*). After a while, however, the increased stretching upon the tight structures of the lower back, which are also likely to be present with EDP, would begin to cause pain.

So what is the best way to sit?

This can vary depending upon the type of pain you are suffering with. However, I will explain here what I feel is generally the best position for you to sit in:

Relaxed Upright: The first thing is to make sure your back is upright, in that you are maintaining the natural lordosis of the lumbar spine. I am going to emphasise the *relaxed* part of this statement though, as it is important your back is not stiff and regimental in nature. If you try to sit bolt upright it is likely to result in further aches and pains, especially if you are suffering with EDP.

Supported: It is important your back, and in particular your lower back, is supported. The best way to achieve this is to make sure that when you sit down, your bottom is pushed back into the chair and not sitting a few inches (or more) away from it. When you have adopted this position, simply sit yourself back into the chair, so that the back of the chair is supporting your whole back.

There is nothing wrong with allowing yourself to relax back into the chair, *as long as your back is supported.* It is when your bottom is not into the back of the chair and you relax back that problems can begin. This will be because your lower back would then curve into the space created between your back and the chair, therefore being unsupported and losing its natural lordotic curve…a recipe for aggravating low back pain and sciatica.

In addition to making sure your bottom is pushed back into the chair, you may also require some kind of extra lumbar support, such as a small, rolled-up towel. Even if your bottom is pushed right back into the chair, the chair may be one where your lower back does still not receive adequate support. Therefore, your lower back will still tend to curve a little into the chair, losing its natural lordosis as mentioned in the previous paragraph. By placing a small support in your lower back, this will help to support, and therefore maintain, the natural curve of your lower back.

Some people have said to me they prefer to sit on the edge of the chair and sit in a relaxed upright position themselves, without any support. This may well be okay, but the chances are this will only be for a short time; after this the stabilising muscles may begin to fatigue a little and the body will then start to recruit other muscles to help support the back, whose primary role is not stability, but movement.

When this occurs, the tendency is for the natural lordosis to become increased as these other muscles begin working harder. This can place too much stress across the facet joints of the lumbar spine and therefore aggravate pain, especially if you are suffering with EDP. Alternatively, as the stability muscles begin to fatigue, the natural lordosis may be lost in the opposite direction as you begin to 'slump' (flexion of the lumbar spine) and therefore potentially aggravate FDP.

> *Ultimately, I feel it is best to push your bottom into the back of your chair, place a suitable support in the small of your low back and then 'relax' into the chair. You should then be in a position where you are relatively upright, but feel relaxed and supported.*

Duration: I suggest the longest you sit without standing up is approximately 15-20 minutes. However, this does not mean you then have to stand or walk around for another 15-20 minutes. As I have mentioned before, sitting tends to place a flexion stress across your spine, whereas standing and walking are naturally upright postures. By standing yourself up every 15-20 minutes you will be removing this flexion stress and replacing it with a nice neutral position. I am more than happy if you only stand and walk around for 30 seconds or so, as long as you break your sitting posture.

I appreciate that if you are sitting down and engrossed in a TV programme, working at a computer or in conversation, before you know it an hour or more may pass without you even noticing. As a little reminder, I would suggest that, if it is the TV you are watching, you take a break every time the adverts come on. Alternatively, I have had some patients tell me they set the timer on their cooker for twenty minutes, and therefore every time it goes off they have to stand and walk a little in order to reset it!

I encourage the need to break any prolonged sitting posture because the longer you stay sitting in one position, the more flexed your posture is likely to become and therefore the more stress you will be placing upon your lower back. By repeatedly standing up, you will be intermittently removing these stresses and therefore encouraging further healing to take place.

As always, I shall leave it up to you with regard to how you sit. What I have written is, in theory, the best way to sit and look after your back. We are all different, however, and, particularly if you are suffering with EDP, you may find you prefer to sit not quite so upright, maybe even a little slumped. Within reason I do not mind this; however, I would still strongly recommend that even in this position, you place some kind of support behind your lower back, as it is always important that your low back is supported when sitting. Also, make sure you stand yourself up for breaks every fifteen to twenty minutes.

How Sitting Can Aggravate Your Pain

Below, I will give three different examples of how sitting can aggravate your pain, beginning with the obvious, i.e. sitting in a chair.

IN A CHAIR

This definitely tends to aggravate FDP. This is because sitting tends to be a naturally flexed posture, therefore encouraging flexion of the lower back. As we sit, even if in a firm upright chair, the lumbar spine will tend to flex. The softer and lower the chair, the more flexed the lumbar spine will become.

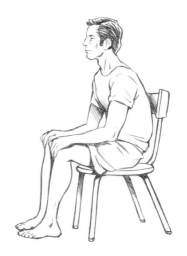

Flexion of the lumbar spine is likely to increase further if you rest your feet up on some kind of foot stall or chair. This is because as your feet are resting upon the stool, your legs will tend to pull your pelvis forward away from the back of the chair, thereby decreasing its support. This in turn will lead to the lumbar spine itself curving into the space created between your pelvis and the back of the chair. Also, if your legs are out straight, this will have a tendency to stretch/pull on the Hamstring muscles and sciatic nerve. If these structures are tight and/or sensitive, there is a likelihood your pain will be aggravated.

Finally, if the seat of a chair is quite deep, this too can make it difficult to place your pelvis into the back of the chair, once again making it difficult to provide your lower back with support. Remember, the closer your pelvis is to the back of the chair, especially if supported by some kind of lumbar support, the less likely your lumbar spine is to go into flexion and therefore the less stress there will be upon your back.

If sitting on a settee is aggravating your pain, I strongly suggest you try sitting in a firmer chair, maybe a dining or computer chair, and then use a rolled-up towel placed in the small of your lower back for support. This may seem a nuisance, but it is only a temporary action I ask you to take, just in order for the body to begin healing itself and therefore become stronger.

As it becomes stronger you are likely to find your back will be able to tolerate sitting on the settee again. If that is the case, feel free to begin to do so, although I would still like you to bear in mind the general principles given in this section with regard to sitting.

> *A little bit of an aside, but if sitting is an aggravating factor for your pain and you are having problems with your sleep and/or having pain and stiffness first thing in the morning, make sure you are not sitting for too long, or in a poor posture, during the few hours before you go to bed. A common complaint I see is that, as a result of excess sitting in the evening, people have a disturbed sleep or stiff and sore back in the morning. See the chapter,* **Practical Advice: Do Not Replace Your Bed** *with regard to this, and do not fall into the trap of replacing your bed prematurely.*

AT THE COMPUTER

The tendency here is not to slump back into the chair as we would do in a soft settee, but rather to lean forward towards the computer (as shown on the opposite page), thus resulting in a similar flexed posture.

When sitting at a computer, you should make sure you are in a relaxed upright posture with the screen directly in front of you at eye level.

Remember the principles given earlier, starting on **page 130** under *'So what is the best way to sit?'* When sitting for any activity, as a rule of thumb, these principles apply and will encourage you to sit in the best way to facilitate healing and therefore rid yourself of the pain you are suffering.

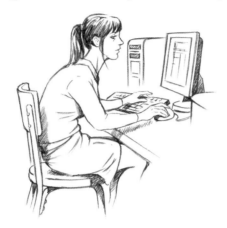

DRIVING

Although not necessarily soft, car seats are typically low and often slope backwards. This again creates flexion in the lumbar spine. If the car permits, it may be best to sit on a pillow or a wedge-shaped pillow in order to bring your hips at least level, if not slightly above, your knees. As mentioned previously with regard to sitting in a chair, you are also likely to benefit from some kind of lumbar support. Although most cars now have lumbar supports built into the seats, in my experience they are not great. If you feel your back needs further support, use something extra such as a lumbar support or a rolled-up towel.

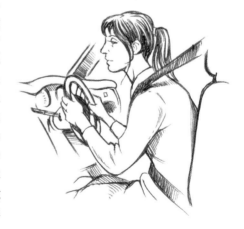

In some respects sitting in a car is like being at a computer, in that our hands are placed out in front of us on the steering wheel, therefore encouraging us to flex forward. I find the best way to counter this is to make sure that every time you sit in the car to make a journey, you sit in a relaxed, upright and supported posture as previously discussed.

Once you are comfortable, adjust your rear-view mirror so you can see clearly out of the rear window. I can almost guarantee by the time you are a few minutes down the road, if you look in the rear-view mirror again you will see about half of the ceiling of your car as well. The reason for this is that you have started to slump forward.

When you notice this, ***do not alter the mirror!*** Instead, alter your posture as it is this which has changed. Continue to correct your posture whenever you begin to see part of the ceiling while looking in the mirror.

Make sure you adjust the mirror to its correct position whenever you embark on a new journey. This is because we lose a little height as the day progresses and therefore the correct position for the mirror in the morning will be slightly different to the correct position for your last journey of the day.

As an aside, you may well notice as you take the above into account, it will help ease any neck pain you may be experiencing, as well as your low back pain or sciatica!

Just before we finish this section, I need to highlight the many different ways there are of sitting down. You may be sitting in a low chair, high chair, soft chair or a firm chair. It may be with your feet flat on the floor or they may be up on a stool. You may be sitting in the corner of the settee or on the floor. If on the floor it may be with your back against a settee with your legs flat out in front of you or maybe with your legs crossed; then again you may not be leaning against anything.

I am sure you understand where I am going with this. Sitting is not simply sitting. You need to take a step back and think about the exact way you are sitting and the effect that particular position may be having upon your back.

SIT TO STAND

This movement can aggravate either FDP or EDP for different reasons. With regard to FDP, the pain may arise due to the disc being 'squeezed' too much too soon as you stand up. However, if you are suffering with EDP, you may feel pain when performing this movement as a consequence of overstretched muscles or soft tissues. If I can refer you back to **Step Four: *How to Diagnose Your Pain*** you will find a full and thorough explanation as to why both FDP and EDP can give you pain during this movement.

STANDING

Standing is not just one simple posture we adopt, there are many ways this can have different influences on your pain. I will explain three of them as follows:

Standing

In its purist form, standing is literally that: a nice upright position with the core stability muscles holding the back in a nice neutral posture.

Pelvic Tilt

This usually occurs where the pelvis is being tilted anteriorly and is a result of weak core stability muscles, typically the abdominals, as well as tight muscles, usually the Quadriceps and Iliopsoas. It is the position where it feels like there is an increased 'arch' (lordosis) in your lower back and would tend to aggravate people suffering with EDP. This type of posture is explained in more detail in the chapter, **Learning Zone: *Why Muscles are the Key***

Factor in Eliminating Your Pain, under the sections Abdominals, and Quadriceps and Iliopsoas. Exercises given to counter this are provided during **Step Six:** *Move Forward with Stretching Exercises* and **Step Seven:** *Move Forward with Core Stability Exercises*.

Leaning forward

Classic examples of this would be shaving, putting on makeup, cleaning your teeth, cooking and washing up at the sink. I have often treated patients who have told me that standing up aggravates their pain when they are referring to these kind of activities. Although it is standing up, there tends to be a flexion stress across the back and it would therefore tend to aggravate someone with FDP, although, as has been explained before, prolonged flexion can also aggravate EDP if there are tight muscles present.

With many of these positions, such as cleaning your teeth, shaving and putting on your makeup, these activities do not need to be performed while stooped forward. If this is the case, then obviously stand more upright when performing them.

For other activities it may not be quite so simple; for these, I would suggest standing up little and often in order to break the prolonged static posture.

No matter what position you are in when standing, if you stand for any length of time without moving, it can aggravate any type of low back pain or sciatica. I'm sure you can anticipate what I am about to say now… if this is the case, do not stand for that long without moving around a little. Remember, the human body likes movement, it is not made to be stuck in one position for prolonged periods of time.

WALKING

I refer to walking as an upright posture. However, it can readily create increased extension of the lumbar spine. The reason for this is that every time we take a stride forward with one leg, the stance leg we 'leave behind' has a degree of extension at the hip. If there is decreased core stability about the lower back along with tight muscles present, in particular the hip flexors (see the chapter, **Learning Zone:** *Why Muscles are the Key Factor in Eliminating Your Pain*), there is a fair chance the lower back will begin to over-extend as well. Therefore, if you are suffering with EDP it should come as no surprise that walking may aggravate your pain due to this increased extension in the lumbar spine.

If this is true for yourself, you will also benefit from the stretches given for Quadriceps and Iliopsoas in **Step Six:** *Move Forward with Stretching Exercises* as well the core stability exercises given in **Step Seven:** *Move Forward with Core Stability Exercises.*

As always, I'm afraid there is an exception to the rule and this is where there are very tight soft tissues present, in particular, the Hamstrings muscles and the nervous system (namely the sciatic nerve).

The Hamstring muscles travel from the bottom part of the pelvis and pass down the leg to attach just below the knee, as shown in the chapter, **Learning Zone:** *Your Lower Back and Sciatic Nerve.* The sciatic nerve is formed from nerve roots that leave the lumbar spine and sacrum. It then passes through the buttock area and Hamstring muscles as it passes down the back of the leg.

Every time you stride forward with one leg, if your Hamstrings/sciatic nerve are tight, you will be pulling slightly on these structures. From the perspective of the Hamstrings, this will tug on the bottom part of the pelvis which in turn will encourage a posterior rotation/tilting backward force upon the pelvis. This can therefore aggravate the pain experienced by someone suffering with FDP.

In addition to this, the tugging on these tight structures can also lead to the sciatic nerve being irritated. Wherever there is the greatest degree of tension upon the sciatic nerve, this is likely to be where the pain or discomfort itself is perceived. If this tension is created primarily about the nerve roots from where the sciatic nerve originates, the chances are the pain will be felt in the lower back. However, the pain may also be felt further down the sciatic nerve if excess tension is felt there, for example in the buttock or back of the leg.

There can also be referred pain from the original source of stress upon the sciatic nerve, especially if it is the nerve roots which have become inflamed.

In such circumstances, pain can be felt anywhere along the length of the sciatic nerve and its branches, from the lower back down to the foot.

> *It is also possible to experience pain only in the leg/foot and not in the back or buttock area. If this is the case, it is nothing to worry about. The pain is still likely to have its source in the lower back or buttock region and it will be treated exactly the same as any other pain in or from the back.*

I should add, however, if you can walk pain-free, no matter how short a distance, it is important you should do so regularly. During any activity you perform, you will be working the core stability muscles of your lower back and pelvis, and the more you work them the stronger they will become. Therefore, if you can walk for say, five minutes, with no problems, I would encourage you to go for regular five minute walks. As you do so, along with performing the appropriate exercises provided in this book, you will find the distance you can walk pain-free for increases over time. Remember though, do not get carried away and begin to walk through pain: all exercise must be pain-free.

JOGGING/RUNNING

Allow me to refer you to the previous section on walking, as the principles that apply there stand true for jogging as well, in particular, the first example of the back tending to over-extend itself due to weak core stability muscles and/or tight hip flexors. Consequently, the recommended chapters given under the previous section for walking (**Step Six:** *Move Forward with Stretching Exercises* for stretches of the Quadriceps and Iliopsoas muscles, as well the core stability exercises given in **Step Seven:** *Move Forward with Core Stability Exercises*) also apply. It is likely if walking increases your pain, running will aggravate it even more so, as there is greater movement and therefore greater stresses taking place across your lower back.

Just as I mentioned previously under walking, if you can jog/run for a short distance with no problems at all, but after this time your pain sets in, it does not mean you cannot run at all. Feel free to perform regular, short distance runs.

During any activity you perform, you will be working the core stability muscles of your lower back and pelvis, and the more you work them the stronger they will become. Therefore, if you can jog for, say, ten minutes with no problems at all (both while jogging and afterwards), I would encourage you to go for regular ten-minute jogs. As you do so, along with performing the appropriate exercises provided in this book, you will find the distance you can run pain-free increases with time. Remember though, do not get carried away and begin to run while feeling pain; all exercise must be pain-free.

LYING

Now this really does depend upon which position you lie in. I am going to explain four typical positions: Side Lying, Prone Lying, Supine Lying and Crook Lying.

Side Lying

If you are lying on your side, there are still three variations of how you can do this:

KNEES UP TO CHEST/FOETAL POSITION

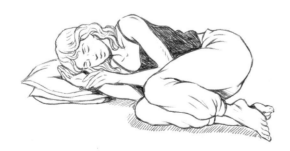

If you are lying in the foetal position, it is more likely to aggravate a FDP back problem and ease an EDP back problem. This is because lying in this position tends to 'flex' the lower back. Therefore, by flexing the lumbar spine you are stretching out the posterior aspects of the back. This may therefore encourage the bulging of a disc (aggravating FDP) yet separate the facet joints (easing EDP).

SIDE LYING WITH YOUR TOP LEG FORWARD AND DOWN

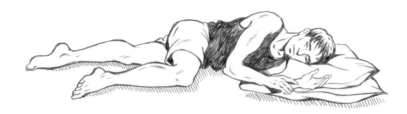

This is a position we typically end up in when lying on our side, even if we started in the foetal position. This position can be painful for either FDP or EDP, especially if there are tight muscles about the lower back/buttock region.

In this position, the top leg tends to drop forward and down over the bottom leg, which in turn causes the pelvis to be rotated forward and down. This will then place a high degree of stress across the lower back and also stretching on the muscles across the back/buttock region, especially if the Gluteal muscles are tight.

SIDE LYING WITH PILLOWS FOR SUPPORT

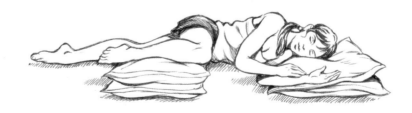

In this position you may be laying on either side, but with the bottom leg straight and top leg supported by pillows. The top leg should be roughly parallel with the bed. By lying in this position, the bottom leg, being straight, is helping to maintain a neutral position for the lower back.

However, by supporting the top leg with pillows, you will be preventing the pelvis from being dragged forward and down by the weight of the leg as described previously with **Side lying with your top leg forward and down**. This also helps to maintain the neutral position of the spine.

As a rule of thumb, this last position tends to be comfortable for both FDP and EDP. A similar position can be adopted whereby a pillow or two is placed in-between the legs instead of having the bottom leg straight. Personally, I feel it is better to keep the bottom leg straight as initially described. However, as always, find the best position for yourself.

Prone Lying

In this position the laws of gravity and natural shape of the spine encourage extension of the lower back. This will therefore force the facet joints together and aggravate EDP.

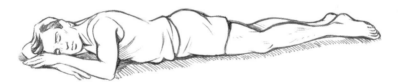

However, by adopting this position, it will help manoeuvre any herniated discs towards their intended position (as described in **Step Four: *How to Diagnose Your Pain***), and therefore may help ease FDP.

If you have a significant disc bulge, then prone lying itself may pinch the disc too much, too soon. This will, therefore, mean prone lying is an aggravating position as it is likely to further inflame the disc. If this is the case, lying with a pillow or two under your stomach usually helps decrease the degree of extension being placed upon the spine and, therefore, tends to feel more comfortable. If this helps, try lying like that for a while and then, as your pain improves, remove the pillows as appropriate.

Supine

As a rule of thumb, this should help ease EDP and aggravate FDP for the opposite reasons to that of prone lying. This is because the laws of gravity will encourage the lower back to sink into the bed/towards the floor, i.e. relative flexion.

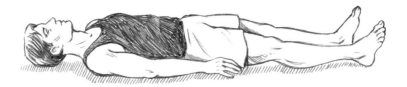

However, it is not always the case. As we are lying in this position, especially if there is decreased stability of the lower back/pelvis and/or tight hip flexors, the pelvis tends to tilt anteriorly (see the chapter, **Learning Zone: *Why Muscles are the Key Factor in Eliminating Your Pain***). This in turn creates extension of the lower back and will, therefore, potentially aggravate an EDP back problem as well and ease a FDP one.

Crook Lying

This tends to be a better position than supine if you are to lie on your back. With this position, common sense tends to prevail in that the laws of gravity do play a role and encourage a flattening of the lower back. The reason this is sometimes more comfortable than supine lying is because your legs are bent at the hips. This takes some of the stretch from the hip flexors, therefore resulting in the back not being placed into relative extension.

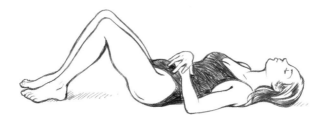

Consequently, this position will tend to ease EDP and aggravate FDP. If you have found this position is better than supine lying, there is a reasonable chance your hip flexors are tight and you have decreased core stability. Therefore, it is important to check these and carry out any appropriate exercises (see **Step Six:** *Move Forward with Stretching Exercises* and **Step Seven:** *Move Forward with Core Stability Exercises*). If you do not like lying in this position with your legs bent, try placing your legs a little flatter but with some pillows underneath your knees.

HOUSEWORK

Unfortunately, this is likely to be the scourge of much low back pain and sciatica, as housework activities are not only typically flexed postures, but they tend to be held for long periods as well. Typical examples are as follows:

Vacuuming and Ironing

These tend to be prolonged flexed postures. Try to avoid these as much as possible while your body is healing itself. If it is not possible to avoid them, modify them instead. For example, when vacuuming use your hips and knees a little more instead of bending forward with your back and looking down at the floor all the time.

When ironing, have the board as high as is possible. If you can have it no higher, maybe try ironing in an upright, relaxed and supported sitting position. With regard to this latter point, most patients find this difficult and do not like it. Give it a go though, as it does work for some people.

If it's impossible to avoid these activities and you are modifying them to the best of your ability, it is still a good idea to break up the activity into small manageable parts. For example, little and often. Maybe iron a little bit each day, say, for only 10 to 15 minutes at a time. Maybe vacuum just one room a day or one room at a time while resting in between.

Making Beds / Cleaning the Bath

These tend to be very flexed postures which, with regard to cleaning the bath, can be held for a relatively prolonged period of time. Unfortunately, they are difficult activities to modify, therefore do your best to avoid them or get someone else to help!

Cooking / Washing Up

I've had many patients refer to these as simply standing up. Although it is, it usually involves slight flexion of the lower back where we are bent over a little. Equally important though, is the fact that these positions tend to be held for prolonged periods of time. Therefore it should come as no surprise to learn that they usually aggravate FDP. Although do remember, prolonged stretching of the back can also aggravate EDP as well.

The best way to modify these activities, is to perform them on as high a work top as is possible when cooking/preparing dinner. Also, maybe try placing a washing-up bowl on top of an upside down one when washing up. Once again give yourself a break little and often.

CLEANING TEETH/SHAVING /PUTTING ON MAKEUP

These are very similar to the previous example, in that prolonged flexion is involved. The good thing here is that there is no need to carry out these activities bent forward. Stand up straight while performing them.

The list goes on and on and I'm sure you can think of many more… cleaning floors, dusting, filling and emptying the washing machine/dishwasher, etc. All of these involve degrees of flexion which, even if not painful when carrying out one particular activity, can build up over a period of time throughout the day. It really is important to try and avoid these activities as much as possible or at least modify them and break them up into smaller manageable parts.

GARDENING

This is very similar to housework, in that it tends to be a flexed posture which is adopted and also held for prolonged periods of time. Therefore, my advice is very similar. Temporarily avoid it if possible. If not, maintain a neutral posture as much as possible and give yourself breaks little and often.

If your pain is one that is better in the morning, but gets worse as the day goes on, there is a fair chance it is repeated activities like those mentioned in this chapter that are having a cumulative stressful effect on your lower back and/or sciatic nerve. This is because your back has had a chance to rest and therefore repair itself overnight, but as you apply further stresses across it with your day-to-day activities it will tend to aggravate your pain again. After a night's sleep, however, your body has begun to heal itself and therefore feels better.

*I strongly suggest you read the following chapter, **Practical Advice: How Recognising Daily Patterns of Pain Will Help Cure Your Pain** for further information on this and other daily patterns of pain.*

Practical Advice:

*How Recognising Daily Patterns of
Pain Will Help Cure Your Pain*

ARE THERE ANY DAILY PAIN PATTERNS WHICH MAY HELP ME RESOLVE MY PAIN?

Yes, there can be. I will explain the typical daily pain patterns now. You may well notice I make reference to some of these elsewhere within this book, relative to the particular aggravating/easing factor.

Mornings are always worse; the pain then gets better and better as the day goes on.

With this scenario, you definitely need to look at the position you are sleeping in. Typically, if you are waking with increased pain and stiffness first thing in the morning, the likelihood is that it is the position you are sleeping in or what you were doing during the late afternoon/evening that is resulting in your mornings being more painful. However, if it is only mornings that are your problem, I would be looking more at the position you are sleeping in. This is because if your late afternoon/evening activities were having an influencing factor on your morning pain, it is likely your pain would at least become a little more uncomfortable during the evening or on retiring to bed. Do not discount the evening, however, I am simply saying the likelihood is it is your sleeping position that is the problem. I strongly suggest you read the following chapter, **Practical Advice: *Do Not Replace Your Bed.***

Mornings are always worse, the pain then eases as the day goes on until the evening, when my pain starts to increase again.

I alluded to this in the previous daily pattern. If I start from the morning where you are feeling increased pain, once again we are looking at two potential factors: the position you were sleeping in and what you were doing in the late afternoon/evening. Your sleeping posture may be a problem, but it is also likely to be the things you have been doing prior to going to bed which are playing a role, especially as it is in the evening when your pain begins to increase again.

One good rule of thumb is to ask yourself *"Is it pretty much the same every morning or does it vary from day to day?"* If the answer to this question is that it varies from day to day, I would be inclined to analyse in particular what it is you have been doing before going to bed (late afternoon/evening) as the chances are you sleep in a similar position every night.

If, however, mornings are pretty much the same every day, then it will be a process of elimination with regard to your evening activities and/or your sleeping position which may be the problem.

Without wanting to sound too judgemental, I would particularly look at what you were doing during the few hours before going to bed, as it is during this time that your pain begins to worsen.

If, during the evening, you are performing an activity or you are in a posture which you know may aggravate your pain, there is every chance your back will tighten up overnight in response to this. This will consequently lead to it feeling particularly stiff and painful first thing in the morning.

Once you are up, however, and become more active during the day, your pain feels a lot better...until the evening when you start to relax, and potentially aggravate your pain again. If this is a pattern you recognise, there is every chance your pain is very 'posturally related' in that it likes activity, i.e. being up and about, but does not like being stuck in one position, usually sitting. Break this pattern and you will begin to reduce the stresses being placed upon your back in the evening. This will result in you feeling more comfortable during this time.

As a consequence of your pain being aggravated less during the evening, your back will have less cause to tighten up overnight and therefore more healing will take place. Finally, because it has not tightened up overnight and healing has taken place, your pain will be more comfortable in the morning. You should then start to see a positive cycle, with your pain progressively improving, as opposed to a negative cycle where your pain fails to improve or gets worse.

I once treated a patient who complained of a similar pattern to that just given, i.e. worse in the morning, better during the day but worse again in the evening. However, with this particular patient, she stated her pain was not that bad every morning and evening. On further questioning it became apparent that her pain was better the morning after she performed an evening shift at work. Her job was a fairly active one where she never sat down for too long, and on returning from work she usually had a quick sit down, cup of tea and was then off to bed.

On the other hand, when she wasn't at work, she would spend much of the evening sitting down watching TV. I explained to her it was likely the activity her back was encountering while at work was better for her, and that if she was to keep a little more active during the evenings when she was not at work, the subsequent mornings should improve also. She tried this, simply by standing up and having a little walk up and down her living room every 20 minutes or so, and her pain did begin to improve. This, along with an exercise programme, was enough to free this patient of pain.

Mornings are great; it is just as the day progresses that my pain becomes worse, until the evening when it starts to settle down again.

This may sound like I am stating the obvious, but it is what you are doing during the day that is aggravating your pain! When you rest in the evening your low back pain/sciatica begins to recover. Come the morning, after a night's sleep, your pain will have recovered well and you have no, or very little, problems at all. However, as soon as you get into your day-to-day activities, your pain begins to increase again.

Whatever your day involves, whether it is at work or at home, you need to look at what it is you are doing with your back in order to elicit the specific postures/activities which are causing you pain. When you have worked these out, you then need to avoid or modify these activities as much as possible. I appreciate this can be easier said than done, but it will help you on the road to recovery. I suggest you read the previous chapter, **Practical Advice:** *The Influence of Regular Day-to-day Activities on Your Pain.*

In addition to this, it would also be a good idea to take a look at what it is you are doing during the evening, as your back obviously likes this and consequently your pain is easing. Therefore, there is every chance you may be able to identify an easing factor for your pain as well.

Mornings are great; it is just as the day progresses that my pain becomes worse until I go to bed.

This is very similar to the above daily pain pattern only this time what you are doing in the evening is still aggravating your pain. Look for any similarities in what you are doing during the day, relative to the evening. It could be that you have aggravated your pain so much that even if you are doing the correct things for it during the evening, there is not enough time for your pain to recover. If this is the case, it is likely your pain is in a reasonably acute stage. I would definitely refer you to **Step Two:** *How to STOP Acutely Inflamed Pain* in order to settle things down a little.

Having said that, a positive to take from this pattern, is that although you are consistently aggravating your pain during the day, your back is also strong enough to recover very well overnight to enable you to have very little or no pain in the morning. This is a good sign, and if you can exclude the aggravating factors during the day, the healing process taking place overnight should also extend further and further into the day. I would anticipate from this that as soon as you eliminate these aggravating factors, your back will recover well and also fairly rapidly.

It's just sleeping which is my problem, apart from that I have no pain at all.

This is similar to *"Mornings are always worse; the pain then gets better and better as the day goes on".* whereby the main problem appears to be the position you are sleeping in. The difference here, I would say, is that your pain is very mechanical in its nature. I say this because although you are probably sleeping in a position that is aggravating your pain and therefore waking you at night, it is not enough to unsettle your back and make it stiff and sore first thing in the morning. I would definitely suggest you read the following chapter, **Practical Advice:** *Do Not Replace Your Bed* to find an alternative way of sleeping.

It is important not to be complacent, however, and not take note of what you are doing late evening/before going to bed. Just as I explained with *"Mornings are always worse; the pain then gets better and better as the day goes on".* it is unlikely this is the case, as you would probably notice an increase in your pain towards the end of the day. However, as I said, you should not be complacent; therefore have a look at your evening activities as well.

There is no pattern at all; my pain is just there all the time.

If this is the case, you still need to analyse things. Even though the pain may be constant, it is still likely there are some activities or postures that make it a little worse, as well as some that make it a little easier. If you can find them, avoid the former and encourage the latter.

One thing is for sure, if your pain is constant, it is likely to be in an acutely inflamed state, therefore you definitely need to read **Step Two: *How to STOP Acutely Inflamed Pain***.

There is no pattern at all, every day is different.

Under these circumstances I would ask you to keep some kind of diary as to what it is you are doing each and every day. It is very rare that pain will be aggravated by certain activities one day and yet the next day those exact same activities do not increase your pain at all. Note down what it is you are doing each day, from morning through to night.

Also, give yourself some kind of pain rating around the morning time, middle and end of the day for the previous 8 hours or so, maybe from 0–10 (0 being no pain and 10 being the worst pain you could ever imagine). When you have done this for several days, look back over your notes and try to elicit any kind of pattern between your pain rating and the activities you were performing that day. I'm not going to say 100 per cent categorically that there is always a pattern, but without doubt there nearly always is.

BOOM AND BUST

One really important thing to add with regard to there being no pattern to your pain is that it is not uncommon for bad days to follow good and vice versa. The reason for this is what I refer to as a '***Boom and Bust***' pattern; the typical scenario is as follows:

The individual concerned may be having a really good day and therefore they think…

> *"My pain feels okay today; I'll take advantage of it and do the things I cannot do when my pain is bad."*

This may be housework or gardening, for example, as these are typical activities which aggravate low back pain or sciatica. They will then spend the day cramming in all the things their pain does not normally allow them to do and then – surprise, surprise – either later that day or the following day their pain has increased untold amounts again, so much so they have to 'take it easy' for a while, i.e. perform only easing factors and not aggravating ones.

After taking it easy for a day or so (performing easing factors), their pain begins to feel better, so what happens? They get stuck into all the jobs again which they have not been able to do for the last few days, i.e. the ones which aggravate their pain, so what happens again…? I'm sure you can see how this cycle continues…and you may well recognise it!

Like any vicious cycle, we need to cut into this classic Boom and Bust cycle somewhere, let's say during a good day. With regard to pain, I am a great believer in the adage that we reap what we sow. Therefore, with regard to this good day, I am going to say there is a fair chance this individual will be having a good day as a result of he or she doing the right things for their pain. The problem here is that rather than think…

> ### *"My back feels really good at the moment, whatever it is I have been doing I am going to carry on doing as it is helping." (i.e. easing things),*

they think

> ### *"My back feels really good at the moment, I am going to do all the things that my pain will not normally let me do." (i.e. aggravating things).*

If we can stop at this point and say to ourselves, *"My back feels really good at the moment, whatever it is I have been doing I am going to carry on doing it, as it is helping,"* we will then begin to break this vicious cycle and instead create a positive one, where the back continues to go from strength to strength.

As your back continues to get stronger, you will find you can slowly but surely introduce what were your aggravating factors. Only this time, as your back is stronger, it will be able to tolerate them.

Therefore, if you feel there is no pattern at all to your pain, be aware of this Boom and Bust cycle and make sure you are not a victim. Remember, if you are having a good day, the chances are that this is a result of what you have been doing to your back; therefore, do not change it, keep it the same. If you do this, your pain should continue to improve.

Finally, if you have been analysing things as much as possible and you are absolutely sure there is no pattern at all to your pain, and it is getting no better even after carrying out the principles of this book, pay a visit to your GP. There is a chance it may not be mechanical in nature and therefore it is best to have it assessed by a health professional.

The following chapter, **Practical Advice: *Do Not Replace Your Bed* is** written with the aim of preventing you from unnecessarily replacing your bed. If you are not getting a good night's sleep, or waking with pain and stiffness in the morning, it is more than likely that your bed *is **not*** the problem, but rather what you are doing before you go to bed or the position you are sleeping in that is. You will discover, by reading the following chapter, that a few simple changes can make all the difference to your pain and also save you a lot of money.

Practical Advice:

Do Not Replace Your Bed

There are a few myths I would like to bust with this book, and one that particularly annoys me is that if you have a bad back or sciatica, and especially if you are not sleeping well, you have to replace your bed…and in particularly with an orthopaedic one. Absolute *RUBBISH!*

More often than not, the reason for you not sleeping well will not be due to the bed itself, but rather the position you are sleeping in or what it was you were doing during the few hours before you went to bed.

This chapter follows on well from the previous two, in that although it is not a day-to-day activity as such, it is one we obviously perform 'daily' for approximately six to eight hours, although that may not be the case at the moment if your pain is quite severe.

Once again it boils down to posture and how we need to keep our spine as near to the ideal neutral position as possible, or at least the ideal posture for your particular problem.

Firstly, let's consider whether we are sleeping well or waking well. If you are sleeping fine and waking with no pain, there is no need at all to replace your bed. That may seem obvious, but you'll be surprised at the number of people I have treated who have replaced their bed because they thought (or at least were led to believe) it was the bed that was causing their pain, when in fact it had nothing to do with it.

Having said that, if you are not sleeping well and/or waking with significant pain and stiffness in the morning, there is still a fair chance it is not your bed that is the problem, but what you were doing with your back before you went to bed or while you were in bed.

So once again you need to start asking yourself questions and in particular…

What was I doing during the few hours before I went to bed?

What position was I sleeping in?

If the answer to either of these is a posture or activity that resembles an aggravating activity for your pain, it should come as no surprise you are finding it difficult to get to sleep, waking during the night or waking with increased pain and stiffness in the morning.

Let's use a couple of examples to highlight this point:

If you are suffering with FDP and have spent most of the evening sitting in a chair watching TV, using the computer, performing housework, etc. (i.e. a flexion dominated postures) it is likely that this position has aggravated your pain.

Due to you having aggravated your pain before going to bed, it should come as no surprise if you find it difficult to get comfortable in bed and/ or get to sleep when you retire for the night.

When you finally get to sleep, your back may start aching and therefore wake you at night. This is because sometimes it is not while you are performing an aggravating activity that you feel the pain most, but rather a little while afterwards.

Finally, if your pain has been aggravated and you spend the next few hours in a relatively still position, there is a fair chance your back will tighten up in response to this. Consequently, it will feel stiff and painful first thing in the morning.

To compound this issue, not only may you not be sleeping well and/or waking with increased pain and stiffness, but **night time is prime healing time**. Therefore, if you are aggravating your problem during the night, you are interfering with quality healing time.

Once you have been noting what position you are sleeping in as well as what you are doing before going to bed, you should start to notice a pattern, i.e. aggravating/easing factors. Hopefully, you will know by now what to do with these…

Avoid the aggravating factors

and

encourage the easing factors.

So, therefore, if you were to notice it is always after performing such-and-such an activity that you tend to have a poor night's sleep and/or wake with pain and stiffness in the morning, try avoiding this activity/posture to see if it makes any difference.

The opposite is true too: if you were to have a good night's sleep and/or wake feeling quite mobile the next morning, make a note again of what you were doing the night before and try to encourage that activity. I am asking you to do this as there is a reasonable chance your back liked that particular activity, which is why you felt less pain and stiffness as a result.

SO WHAT POSITION SHOULD I SLEEP IN?

Before I go any further, I want to repeat my philosophy for the whole of this book, and that is you should always listen to your body. What do I mean by that? Well, without sounding too flippant, the best position for you to sleep in is the position in which you get the best night's sleep and wake up feeling the most comfortable in the morning.

I am reinforcing this because if you try any of the positions suggested in this chapter and find your pain gets no better or even worse, try something different. Initially, modify the position in some way, but if that doesn't work change the position completely. Remember, your body will know what it likes best, so listen to it.

With regard to sleeping postures, there are primarily three positions you can adopt.

i)   **Prone**
ii) **Supine**
iii) **On your side**

I shall now go through each of these positions and highlight which type of pain they would typically aggravate or ease.

Prone Lying

Prone lying will tend to aggravate EDP. This is because as you sleep, the laws of gravity (and the give in the bed) will encourage your back to sink into the bed and therefore go into a position of relative extension. This will 'force' the posterior structures of the back, in particular the facet joints, to press against one another and consequently cause pain. Therefore, it should be no surprise that if you are suffering with EDP this can increase your pain while in bed and make it stiff and sore in the morning.

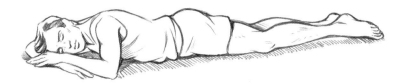

I should also mention that with this position, although in theory it should be good for those suffering with FDP (you will discover it is an early exercise given for FDP in **Step Five: *Getting Moving Again***), you can have too much of a good thing. Therefore, if you were to spend several hours in this position it may also aggravate your pain. In addition to this, it may be that you need to decrease the degree of extension taking place in your back by placing a pillow or two underneath your stomach.

Supine Lying

This position can tend to aggravate either FDP or EDP. The reasons for this are as follows:

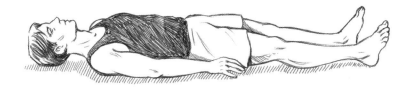

FDP: In this position, the laws of gravity can have the opposite effect to that of Prone Lying, in that it will encourage relative flexion of your lumbar spine, especially if the bed is particularly soft. If you are suffering with FDP and your back is held in relative flexion for most of the night, it should be no surprise it becomes aggravated.

However, this is not always the case. If you are lying on your back with your legs straight and you have weak core stability muscles and/or tight hip flexors, this tightness can result in the pelvis being pulled into anterior rotation and therefore creating relative extension of your lower back (see the chapter, **Learning Zone:** *Why Muscles are the Key Factor in Eliminating Your Pain* where it is discussed under Quadriceps and Iliopsoas as well as Abdominals). If you are suffering with FDP and your back is being held in an extended position, this may actually feel like a reasonably comfortable position.

EDP: As mentioned above under FDP, the laws of gravity can have the opposite effect to that of Prone Lying, in that it will encourage relative flexion of your lumbar spine, especially if the bed is particularly soft. Therefore, if you are suffering with EDP and your back is being held in relative flexion for most of the night, this should feel like a fairly comfortable position.

Once again though, and with reference to the last paragraph under FDP, if you have weak core stability muscles and/or tight hip flexors, the pelvis may be forced into anterior rotation in this position, which is relative extension of the lower back. Consequently, extension of the lumbar spine will tend to aggravate the pain of someone who is suffering with EDP. If supine lying is uncomfortable for this reason, many people prefer to adopt a crook lying position or place some pillows under their knees to try and take the pressure from the tight hip flexors and consequently their lower back.

Side Lying

This can aggravate any type of back problem. When we lie on our side, we tend to adopt one of two positions, either the foetal position or side lying with the top leg across and down.

The foetal position, if you can imagine, is like a sitting position, but on your side. We know that sitting is a flexion-dominated posture therefore this position can either aggravate FDP or ease EDP.

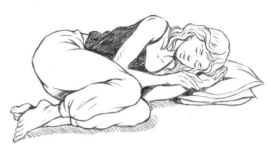

However, the reality is that as we sleep the top leg tends to drop over the bottom leg, as shown below. This puts a rotational strain across the lumbar spine and stretches the soft tissues on the outside of the hip and upper leg, in particular the Gluteal muscles. If the back is held in this twisted position and the soft tissue structures are being stretched for several hours, it should come as no surprise if you have a difficult night's sleep and suffer with pain and stiffness in the morning.

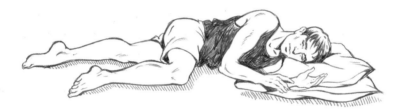

SO WHAT IS THE BEST POSITION THEN?

At this stage it may well appear I am making things difficult, as all of the positions I have discussed above can aggravate either type of pain.

In my opinion, by far the most comfortable position for any type of pain to be sleeping in (although admittedly not always the most practical) is side lying while using pillows to support your top leg (any mothers or pregnant ladies reading this will be familiar with what I am suggesting).

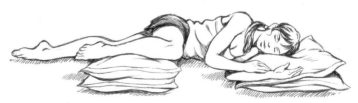

This position is pretty much the same as the second side lying position just discussed. However, as you lie on your side, let's say your left side, keep this bottom leg straight while you bend your right hip and knee, and place it on top of a couple of pillows.

By keeping the bottom leg straight, we are helping to keep the back in a neutral position. However, by supporting the top leg with pillows, we are preventing the pelvis from rolling forward and down, placing the back and soft tissues under less stress than the previous positions.

With regard to the number of pillows needed, I mention two here simply because that is 'about right'. However, it will depend upon the size of your pillows and also the size of your 'hips'. Ultimately though, you need to work it out for yourself depending upon what your pain tells you. In theory, your top leg should be pretty much parallel with the bed itself. My experience tells me, however, most people tend to prefer the top leg to be slightly lower than this…find out what best suits you.

If you find this position impractical to maintain, you may wish to try side lying with some pillows in between your knees. Ultimately, though, remember…

The best position for you is the position in which you sleep best and also wake up feeling most comfortable in the morning!

The following chapter, **Learning Zone: *The Principles of Exercise,*** will outline the main principles upon which the exercises given throughout this book are based. Following this will be **Step Five: *Getting Moving Again.*** The latter chapter will guide you through the best way of further reducing your pain by providing you with the knowledge to self-prescribe an exercise programme suited to your specific diagnosis.

Learning Zone:

The Principles of Exercise

Before you begin prescribing yourself an appropriate exercise programme for your low back pain or sciatica, it is important I explain the main principles upon which to base these exercises. If you bear these principles in mind while carrying out your exercise programme, you will progress well and begin to develop a strong, fit and healthy back, free from pain and equally, if not more importantly, strong enough to resist any potential future episodes of pain.

AGGRAVATING AND EASING FACTORS

Never lose sight of this concept. The reason I am bringing this to your attention yet again is because the same principle applies while you are carrying out any exercises. It does not matter whether you are doing something around the house or performing one of the exercises in this book, an aggravating factor is an aggravating factor. Therefore, if any of the exercises aggravate your pain, ease off.

It is important I emphasise this point, as I have treated many patients who feel the approach of *"No Pain – No Gain"* is an appropriate one to take in order to resolve their pain…it is not. I reinforce my views on the *"No Pain – No Gain"* approach in the final chapter, **Old Wives' Tales**.

However, the opposite is true with regard to easing factors. By this I mean if you find any of the exercises particularly ease your pain, be careful but feel free to perform them more often than I have suggested if you wish. The reason I encourage this, is because if your pain is easing, your body obviously likes what it is you are doing and therefore there is more potential for healing to take place.

If you have not done so already, may I suggested you flick back and read **Step Three:** *How to Optimise Your Body's Healing Potential*, as I elaborate during this chapter why it is so important to listen to the Aggravating and Easing factors that relate to your pain.

I know to a certain extent this may be seen simply as semantics; however, I often refer to the term 'awareness' with regard to how you may feel after exercising. By this, I mean you may have finished exercising and are now 'aware' you have just exercised.

For example, you may be aware that you now have some Hamstring muscles if you have just finished stretching them, but they are not sore or painful. If you notice this after you have exercised, as long as it is only awareness and not painful at all, I do not mind. To me, this is simply the body letting you know it has been worked but it is not really complaining about it. Having said that, I would expect this awareness to be resolved within 20-30 minutes or so.

If this is the case, I would suggest you keep the exercises at exactly the same level. With time you should find you no longer have this awareness after exercising. When this happens and you are finding the exercises quite easy, it's time to step them up a level!

I have presented the exercises within this book in a simple, step-by-step, graded way. By performing them this way, they should all increase the appropriate stresses upon your back as you progress. However, ***listen to your body!*** As you embark upon your exercise programme, one of three things will happen:

➤ Your pain will improve.
➤ Nothing changes; your pain is no better or no worse.
➤ Your pain gets worse.

Your pain will improve

If this is the case, then pretty much keep on doing whatever it is you are doing. Your body likes it and healing is taking place.

I always tend to say there are two ways of telling whether your pain is getting better:

i)   You feel less pain. This may be that you are not feeling the pain as much throughout the day, or you are still feeling it as often, but it is not quite as intense.

ii) How quickly your back recovers to its 'normal' level should you aggravate it. For example, I have had patients say, "I did such and such yesterday and it aggravated my pain, yet within an hour or so it was OK again." When I then ask what normally would have happened, they usually reply something like, "Oh, normally I would have suffered for the rest of the day and woken the next morning with increased pain and stiffness."

If you recognise either of these two, your pain is improving. Your lower back/sciatic nerve is getting stronger and therefore able to tolerate more stress. If this stress is increased above the pain threshold level, it is still strong enough to recover quickly as soon as that same stress has been removed.

On the subject of your pain getting better, I always prefer it when patients tell me they feel their pain is improving more and more as each day passes. This is the best news I can hear, as it tells me that the correct conditions are being set up in order for the body's fantastic healing process to be working each and every day.

Now don't get me wrong, the body does not always heal itself in complete linear fashion, whereby every day is a steady improvement on the one before. There are often a few little peaks and troughs along the way. However, if you can look back over the last few days or weeks and note that steady improvement has taken place, then you are doing pretty much all the correct things in order for your body to be healing itself, therefore carry on doing whatever it is you are doing.

I have treated many patients who have reported that their pain was getting better, but it has now plateaued or maybe even worsened. On further questioning it transpires that as their pain eased, they also eased off on their exercises or begun to perform some activities that used to aggravate their pain. It is important you do not make the same mistake.

> *If you feel your pain is improving, do not rest on your laurels and ease off on the exercises or fall back into bad habits, believing the hard work has been done. The reason your pain is better is because of the things you have been doing, therefore continue to do them until you are 100 per cent better.*

Nothing changes; your pain is no better or no worse

If this is the case and you are confident you have given yourself the correct diagnosis, as well as having worked out the correct exercises to perform, we may have to step things up a bit. I would ask you to increase steadily the number or reps, the intensity of the exercise or the number of times per day you are performing the exercises. These exercises may be the correct ones to do, it's just that you are not doing enough of them or not performing them at the correct intensity.

Alternatively, if you do increase the exercises and there is still no change, move on to the next level available. I would say it is unlikely you have prescribed yourself the wrong exercises with regard to your diagnosis. If this were the case, the likelihood is your pain would not have liked the exercises at all, and as you progressed your pain would have increased.

> *The really important thing I wish to highlight here is that if your pain has reached a plateau, even if it was improving beforehand, the chances are you need to progress further with the exercises. Do not rest on your laurels or be reluctant to continue with them.*

Your pain gets worse

If this is the case it is nothing to worry about, it is just your body telling you that you are overdoing it a bit at this particular time. If you are confident you have given yourself the correct diagnosis and have also worked out the correct exercise programme, it is likely you are trying to do a bit too much, too soon. Therefore, all I would ask you to do is stop performing the exercise and wait for your pain to settle down again…it will.

Once it settles back down to its normal level, leave it half a day or maybe until the next day and then begin exactly the same exercises again. Only this time do not perform quite as many, work them quite as hard or carry them out so many times throughout the day. In other words, ease off a little.

If the exercises still continue to aggravate your pain, I would ask you to ease off once or twice more. If, however, they continue to aggravate, the chances are it is not the correct exercise for you at this time. Stop doing them altogether and look at other exercises to do or just continue with the ones which you know your pain is happy with. It may not be all the exercises that are aggravating it, just one or two of them.

If you have done this but still the exercises continue to aggravate your pain, go back a stage or two with regard to listening to your aggravating and easing factors, making sure you have provided yourself with the correct diagnosis and therefore subsequent exercise programme. It may be you have misdiagnosed your problem, which in turn will result in you carrying out the incorrect exercises.

Once again I need to stress the importance of listening to your body and doing what you feel is correct, whilst also adopting common sense. The reason I say this particularly applies to the stretching exercises, as stretches themselves can feel uncomfortable. I have no problem with this and do not want you to stop stretching simply because you feel some discomfort when performing them.

However, as we have already established, we are all unique individuals and our pain and pain threshold levels tend to vary. What is uncomfortable for one person, may be nothing at all for another and yet very painful to someone else. Therefore, just bear in mind the principles outlined before, and go with whether *you feel* the exercises are aggravating or easing *your pain*.

What we must also bear in mind, with regard to the stretches, is that the tight muscles themselves are likely to be contributing to the pain you are suffering, because they are exerting increased stresses across the structures involved. If you stretch that particular muscle group, this will obviously place further stress across those same structures. This should be no problem at all, as the stretch is only to be held for 20–30 seconds. Nevertheless, this increased stress may still be enough to aggravate your pain. If it does, it is nothing to worry about. Simply ease off, wait for things to settle and then begin them again, but just take it a little easier next time.

> *Having highlighted the best ways to progress their exercises, sometimes patients have attended their physiotherapy appointment with me and remarked the exercises were helping and their pain was getting much better, so they decided to carry out even more of them or increased the intensity. Is that wrong? No way, if you feel the exercises are helping and therefore want to increase them, feel free. Just bear in mind the principles I have just given and if they do begin to aggravate your pain, ease off to the level you know your low back pain/sciatica was happy with.*

HOW MANY EXERCISES SHOULD I PERFORM FROM THOSE GIVEN IN THIS BOOK?

That may be a difficult question to answer. Ideally, I obviously want you to carry out all of those exercises that are addressing the potential cause of your pain. Having said that, there is a possibility that for some of you reading this book, that could be quite a few!

If you have worked out what exercises you feel you need to perform, and you feel there are far too many, I do not mind if you cut them down to about 4-6. If you do not, there is a chance you may find it difficult to put aside the time to perform all of them and therefore end up performing none at all.

If you do choose to reduce them to around 4-6, all I would ask is that as you conquer any of those specific exercises and find them quite easy to perform, replace them with, or just add in, any of the other potential exercises you initially left out. Continue to do this until you have performed and conquered all of the appropriate exercises.

On the other hand, if you are happy to perform more than this, I would definitely encourage you to do so, although be careful not to overdo it.

HOW OFTEN SHOULD I PERFORM THE EXERCISES?

As you read through each chapter that provides you with the appropriate exercises to perform, there will be a schedule given advising you approximately how many repetitions of each should be performed, along with how many sets and times per day. It will be set out in the format given on the following page.

Schedule: A guide as to how you should carry out the given exercises each day.

Repetitions: How many times you perform one particular exercise without a specific stop for a rest, e.g. 10 Repetitions.

Sets: How many times you should carry out each group of repetitions whenever you put time aside to perform the given exercises, e.g. 3 sets.

Times per day: Quite simply how many times to perform the above repetitions and sets per day, e.g. 2 times per day.

For example, a specific exercise may have the following detailed:

SCHEDULE:

Repetitions: 10
Sets: 3
Times per Day: 2

This means I am suggesting you perform the given exercise 10 times (**Repetitions**) in one go before giving yourself a little rest (maybe 30-60 seconds). After that rest, you are to perform the exercise 10 times again and repeat this for a total of 3 times (**Sets**). You then continue on to your next exercise until you finish your programme.

Later in the day you will need to perform the same exercises again, until you have performed them twice throughout the day (**Times per Day**).

I am sure you will be familiar with what I am about to say…the schedule I give is not set in stone, it is up to you to tailor it to meet the demands of your body, i.e. either increase or decrease the exercises depending upon how your pain reacts to those exercises.

One final thing with regard to how the exercises are set out within this book. They are numbered 1), 2), 3), etc. and this is done in an order where number 1) is the easiest and number 3) is the most demanding. Therefore, while performing the exercises, if you feel the one you are carrying out is too easy, simply move forward to the next one, e.g. from 1) to 2). On the other hand, if you are finding a particular exercise too difficult or it is causing you pain, move back down the scale from 2) to 1).

WHAT IF I CAN PERFORM AN EXERCISE BETTER ON ONE SIDE COMPARED TO THE OTHER?

If this is the case, I'd like to ask you to even things up a bit, as it's important we keep as symmetrical as possible. Therefore, if you were performing one of the Leg Slide exercises given in **Step Seven:** *Move Forward with Core Stability Exercises* **(page 243)**, I would suggest you only take each leg as far as your 'worst performing side'. As your worst performing side improves, you should find both sides become equal, in which case proceed as appropriate.

I would say the same principle also applies to any stretches. Therefore, using the Hamstring stretches as an example given in **Step Six:** *Move Forward with Stretching Exercises* **(page 225/226)** feel free to stretch each side out if they both need it. However, try to stretch a little more on the tighter side until both sides are equal. Once again, when they become equal, proceed as appropriate.

IMPROVING TOWARDS BEING PAIN-FREE

My advice throughout this book with regard to the schedules I suggest, is that if you are still suffering with pain, no matter how little, you need to perform the exercises 2-3 times per day, every day. It is important you modify this as appropriate, but by performing them this regularly you will be able to get yourself into a good habit of performing the exercises.

I would also suggest you perform the exercises at specific given times, e.g. just before going to work, when you get in from work, just before dinner, etc. The reason I suggest this is because the likelihood of you doing them increases. Experience tells me that those who set aside a specific time each day to perform the exercises do so with greater regularity than those who just think, 'I need to do them x amount of times each day'. With regard to the latter, there is a fair chance you will begin to put the exercises off and before you know it, it's time for bed and you have performed none.

MY LOW BACK PAIN/SCIATICA IS FEELING QUITE GOOD NOW; I'M FRIGHTENED I'LL AGGRAVATE IT AGAIN IF I PERFORM MORE EXERCISES

I can understand how this can be a dilemma for you, although that doesn't mean I agree. If your pain is feeling better as a result of the exercises you are performing, then I want you to continue exercising until you are 100 per cent free of pain, and probably for a couple of weeks or more after that. If for any reason you have reached a plateau, even if your pain is much better than it used to be, I would strongly recommend you continue exercising, and probably either increase the exercises you are performing or add some new ones; *you will not cause any damage at all if you do this.*

If you are not 100 per cent pain-free, it is likely inappropriate stresses are still being placed across those structures causing you pain, and of equal importance is that the structures concerned are not strong enough to withstand these stresses. These stresses may be a result of what you are doing during your day-to-day activities or because of any tight and weak muscles present. Nevertheless, there are stresses still there which need to be eliminated and therefore you need to address them.

As long as you are careful and slowly introduce new and more challenging exercises, the worse thing that will happen is that your pain will increase a little. If that is the case, do not worry as it will settle down again. Therefore do not be frightened to try.

I suggest you read *Nothing changes; your pain is no better or no worse* on **page 174** of this chapter if you are in this quandary. I say this because I would imagine it is because your improvement has plateaued and you are feeling relatively content with your 'better back'. Try not to be complacent; the aim of this book is to free you of pain completely. Be sensible and always stick to the principles given…but do not give up too early, **you may be missing out on a life free of pain!**

MAINTENANCE PLAN: KEEPING YOURSELF PAIN-FREE

Once you have followed the advice in this book and are no longer suffering pain, I am more than happy for you to begin easing off on your exercises. However, I would first suggest you wait two weeks or so of being *100 per cent pain-free* before you do this. If you have achieved this, feel free to reduce the number of exercises you are performing. Once again there is no right or wrong way of doing this, but I would suggest you initially ease off by way of *'times per day'*, gradually reducing your exercises to once per day.

When you have achieved this, let's say over the course of a week or so, feel free to give every other day a miss and once again see how your pain responds. If during the time you are reducing the frequency of your exercises, you feel your pain begin to rear its ugly head again, simply increase the exercises to the level which you know will ensure it is eliminated.

I suggest you continue to perform the exercises you feel were integral in resolving your pain at least 2 to 3 times per week anyway. This will create an ongoing exercise plan to keep your back at its fighting best.

However, if you decide against this and stop performing the exercises altogether, there is still no reason why your pain should return, providing you are sensible with what you do and how you use your back from day to day.

> *If at any stage, however, your pain does begin to return,* ***immediately*** *re-introduce the exercises and postural advice you began with, which you know will eliminate it again. If your pain does happen to return, re-introducing the same principles that eliminated it in the first place will do so again.*

How anyone responds to reducing their exercise programme varies from person to person. Some people reduce their exercises to zero and never suffer an ache or pain again, whereas others need to perform some degree of exercise a few times per week to maintain a pain-free back and sciatic nerve. Only you will be able to find what suits your pain as you slowly reduce your exercise programme with time.

REVERSING THE CURVE

I just thought I would finish this chapter by explaining the concept I refer to as **'reversing the curve'**.

As highlighted in the chapter, **Learning Zone:** *Why You are Feeling Pain,* tightness or weakness in any muscle group can force the lumbar spine to deviate from its neutral posture, which in turn places increased stresses upon the back, potentially leading to pain. We need to decrease these stresses by addressing the deviation away from the neutral posture and bringing the spine back into its correct alignment.

However, sometimes, in order to reduce as much stress as possible from the lower back, thereby enabling quality healing time, we need not just return the spine to its neutral position, but instead 'reverse the curve'.

For example, if you are suffering with FDP, the chances are it is flexion forces across the posterior aspect of your back that are causing you pain. Therefore we need to extend the lumbar spine. This can be achieved by adopting a prone lying position, as shown on the opposite page.

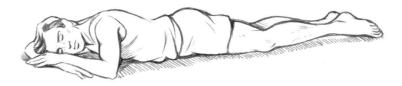

Reversing the Curve…prone lying helps encourage extension of the lumbar spine.

However, if you are suffering with EDP it is likely there are compressive forces about your back, and in particular the facet joints, that are causing you pain. Therefore we need to reduce these stresses by flexing the lumbar spine. This can be achieved by sitting forward and resting on your knees, as shown below.

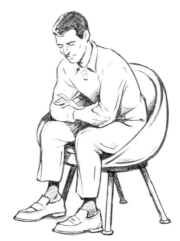

Reversing the Curve…resting forward on your knees helps flex the lumbar spine.

These are only a couple of examples which can be used to 'reverse the curve'. A more detailed explanation of these principles was given in the earlier chapter, **Step Four:** *How to Diagnose Your Pain.*

I am highlighting this within this chapter as it is one of the main principles for the early treatment of FDP and EDP and also because initially it may seem to go against the stated principle of maintaining a neutral spine. We do need to aim for a neutral spine with regard to our day-to-day activities. However, while you are treating your pain and carrying out specific tailored exercises, there is every justification in deviating from then, as long as it is in the correct direction!

Now enjoy the remaining chapters, beginning with **Step Five:** *Getting Moving Again* as you work out a simple but very effective exercise programme for yourself. The exercises you are about to perform will not only alleviate your pain, but also decrease the stresses upon it, making it stronger and therefore reducing the risk of you ever suffering the same pain again.

Step Five:

Getting Moving Again

Okay, for you to begin progressing through this chapter and getting yourself moving again, I am assuming you are now passing through the acute stage of pain, where any kind of movement is difficult, and more towards the mechanical type of pain where movement is easier, although not completely pain-free. This chapter will guide you through the specific exercises for you to choose and tailor-make into a programme which will resolve your pain completely.

IN WHAT ORDER SHOULD I CARRY OUT THESE EXERCISES?

I have set the exercises out 'roughly' in the order which will be best for you to perform, with the exercises becoming slightly more demanding as you progress. However, I can assure you now that you might not advance through them exactly in the order given here. The reason for this is that although you will be suffering pain which falls under the functional diagnosis of either FDP or EDP, there are still likely to be subtle differences from person to person. These differences, although subtle, will enable some people to move on to specific exercises quicker than others. It is for this reason that I am once more going to outline the fundamental theme of this book…

Listen to and be guided by what your body does and doesn't like, remember…

Avoid the aggravating factors

and

encourage the easing factors.

It is imperative you keep this principle a dynamic one. Anything is a potential aggravating or easing factor – a position, a movement or even a prescribed exercise. Whenever you detect one, act accordingly. As I mentioned during **Step Two:** *How to STOP Acutely Inflamed Pain*, aggravating and easing factors can change as your body heals itself, and, if they do, ensure you change your activities and exercises as appropriate.

WHAT IS YOUR DIAGNOSIS?

This is the first thing you need to know before even thinking about progressing through the following exercises. When you have established whether your diagnosis is FDP or EDP, you will then be ready to begin the exercises which follow.

When you feel you can fairly comfortably perform the first two exercises for your given diagnosis, I would ask you also to introduce the ***Stretching and Movement Exercises***, which follow later in this chapter.

As you find these exercises comfortable, we need to move forward once again. Do not waste time by waiting until you can complete all of the exercises given here pain- or stretching-free. Once you feel you are comfortable with your appropriate exercises and are confident they will not aggravate your pain, look to push on. At that stage, I would say you are now progressing really well and would ask you to work your way through the following chapters too:

Learning Zone: *Why Muscles are the Key Factor in Eliminating Your Pain*

This Learning Zone follows this chapter. Here, you will discover how and why muscles can increase inappropriate stresses across your lower back and sciatic nerve, which can ultimately lead to pain.

Step Six: *Move Forward with Stretching Exercises*

This chapter will show you how to stretch any of the muscles given in the previous chapter which you feel are tight and therefore contributing to your pain.

Step Seven: Move Forward with Core Stability Exercises

This chapter will show you how to strengthen the main stabilising muscles for your lower back and pelvis, therefore providing it with greater support, which will assist in eliminating your pain.

The following exercises covered in this chapter are still quite gentle. However, they are effective exercises which will familiarise your back with day-to-day movements again. This will encourage blood flow to the appropriate structures and help decrease any muscle spasm/tightness that may be present.

TREATING FLEXION-DOMINATED PAIN

If you have been analysing your pain and feel it is flexion-type activities that aggravate it, it is likely you are suffering with FDP. Carry out the following exercises to help alleviate your pain.

Extension Exercises for FDP

1) PRONE LYING WITH PILLOWS

Lying on your front, place a pillow or two underneath your stomach to help support your back.

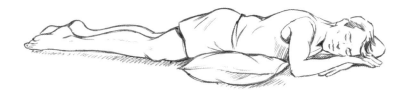

2) Prone Lying

This is quite simply lying flat on your stomach.

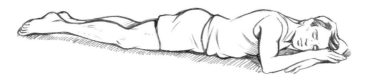

3) Prone Lying on your forearms / in extension

With regard to this exercise, feel free to rest yourself up as high as you are happy to, as long as it does not aggravate your pain.

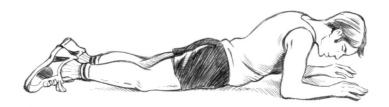

If you get to the stage where you feel you can extend your back more than by just resting on your elbows, maybe push up onto your hands a little as if you are performing a 'top half' press-up, or simply place some pillows or a bean bag under your forearms.

If you have reached this stage, some people find it nice to rest as high up as possible for a little while, let's say 20-30 seconds, and then lower themselves down again for a minute or so followed by propping themselves up again for 20-30 seconds or so and so on. Remember, you work out what works best for you.

Schedule: Exercises 1–3

Repetitions: Lie in this position for approximately 3-5 minutes
Sets: 1
Times per Day: Approximately hourly (if practical)

You may find, when performing the last exercise, that lying in that position may be really comfortable at first, but after a short period of time it becomes uncomfortable. If this is the case, do not stop performing it, rather, lower yourself down a little.

If, however, you lower yourself down so that you are lying in a flat position and the pain is still increased, I suggest it is time for you to finish the exercise for now and get up. Repeat the exercise again after an hour or so.

In general, if you are performing any of the previous exercises and you find them easy, you should progress as appropriate. On the other hand, if you feel they are aggravating your pain, ease back down the scale.

If you are only performing the No 1 exercise *Prone Lying with Pillows* and yet you still feel an increase in your pain, these exercises are not the ones for you *at this particular time*. Stop doing them and think about whether you are truly suffering with FDP.

If you are convinced FDP is the correct diagnosis, still give these exercises a miss for a day or two but in the meantime maybe try some of the resting positions given during **Step Two:** *How to STOP Acutely Inflamed Pain.* When you feel your pain has settled a little, re-introduce exercise No 1 and proceed as appropriate.

If, on the other hand, you feel you may have misdiagnosed your problem, still ease off on the exercises for a while, but when your pain has settled try introducing some of the following exercises for EDP.

The ultimate aim for these exercises is to try and reverse the curve, as discussed in the chapter, **Learning Zone:** *The Principles of Exercise.* The further you can extend your back the better, therefore remember, if the exercise is easy, progress to the stage that you feel is appropriate for you.

What I am about to say may seem to contradict slightly the main principle running throughout this book, namely, that no exercises should aggravate your pain; however, this principle does not fully apply to these exercises. The reason for this is as follows:

The potential areas of pain you perceive in and from your lower back can be described as being more central (towards your back) or more distal (towards your feet). If you are suffering with referred pain from your lower back into the buttock and/or down the leg (i.e. sciatica) as your pain decreases the pain will typically decrease distally first.

For example, you may still be suffering with low back pain but no longer have pain below the knee. I often refer to this as the pain travelling centrally, for obvious reasons. If this does happen, sometimes, although not very often, the pain can increase centrally, i.e. towards or in your lower back.

As long as the distal pains are easing and you feel the pain is 'travelling' towards your lower back, I do not mind.

However, do not grin and bear any increases in your pain; if it becomes too intense or you simply feel you are not benefiting, ease off.

In addition to this, I would also like to note that distally travelling pain is not a particularly good sign. If you are carrying out these exercises and you feel the pain is spreading further down your leg, even if the pain centrally is easing, I would advise you to ease off or stop performing the exercises.

TREATING EXTENSION DOMINATED PAIN

If you have been analysing your pain and feel it is extension-type activities that aggravate it, it is likely you are suffering with EDP. Carry out the following exercises to help alleviate your pain.

With all of these exercises, ideally we are looking for a decrease in pain and/or a feeling of stretching/tightness around the lower back area, although not exclusively there as with some exercises you may find this tightness passes into the buttock region or even down the leg. As long as it is only a feeling of stretching/tightness/pulling, etc., I do not mind: no pain though.

While carrying out these exercises, ensure you gently tighten your stomach muscles while doing so…however, do not hold your breath!

Flexion Exercises for EDP

1) POSTERIOR PELVIC TILT (LYING AND STANDING)

With this exercise, position yourself in crook lying (as shown) and gently flatten your back into the floor.

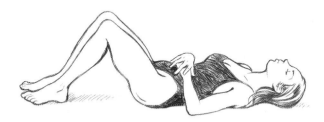

To progress this exercise, stand against a wall (as shown on the following page) with your feet a little away from the wall and your knees slightly bent, then gently flatten your back against the wall.

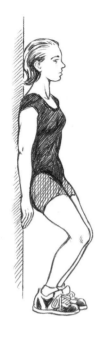

Hold either of these positions for 5-10 seconds and relax. Make sure you do not hold your breath while performing this exercise.

Repetitions: 10
Sets: 3 − 5
Times per Day: 3

This exercise can be surprisingly difficult to perform, as some people find it difficult to isolate lower back from pelvic movements. It can be this inability that is a contributing factor to your pain. The following will provide you with a few 'cues' to use if you are finding either of these exercises difficult. It is assumed you will be performing this exercise in crook lying, as this is the easier of the two positions to carry out this exercise.

i) Flatten your stomach into your lower back/the floor.

As you lie in the crook lying position, imagine you are trying to flatten your stomach downwards as much as you can into your lower back and then the floor.

ii) Rotate your pelvis down into the floor.

As you lie in the crook lying position, place your hands on the outside of your pelvis as shown below. As you attempt to flatten your back, use your hands to encourage your pelvis to rotate backwards towards the floor. This is the motion the pelvis needs to make in order to perform this exercise.

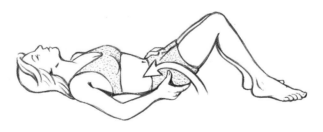

iii) Use your heels and bottom muscles to help out.

As you lie in the crook lying position, gently tighten your buttock/Gluteal muscles while very gently pushing through your heels as you attempt to perform this exercise.

If you are still struggling, feel free to combine any of these cues to assist further.

2) KNEE(S) TO CHEST

For this exercise, lie in the supine position and then gently hug one knee to your chest (holding either behind your knee as shown or on the upper part of your shin). Hold for 5-10 seconds and relax. Repeat with the other leg and then both legs together as shown at the bottom of this page.

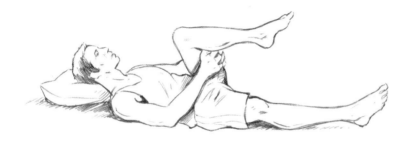

SCHEDULE:

Repetitions: 5
Sets: 3
Times per Day: 3

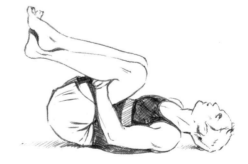

195

3) Four-Point Kneeling Flexion

Placing yourself on all fours, with your hands approximately under your shoulders and knees below your hips, keep your hands in the same position and gently arch your back up towards the ceiling and then lean backwards as if to sit on your heels as shown. We are looking for a stretch around your lower back area. However, you may also feel a stretch further up your back towards your shoulders or down towards your buttocks and even upper leg. If you feel no stretch at all while performing this exercise, keeping your bottom close to your heels, gently stretch your hands further in front of you. Once again we are looking for a stretch in the above mentioned areas.

Hold each stretch for 10-20 seconds and then relax.

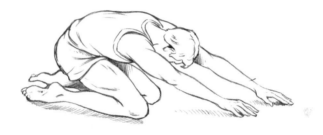

SCHEDULE:

Repetitions: 5
Sets: 3
Times per Day: 3

If you do feel a stretch in your buttock region (Gluteals) it is likely these muscles are also tight, as long as it is only a stretch this is no problem. However, I would suggest you try the Gluteal stretch given on **page 220** in **Step Six: *Move Forward with Stretching Exercises.***

It is important when performing this last exercise to keep the back arched upwards, even if only a small amount. There can be a tendency to allow your back to 'drop down' when performing this exercise. This is exactly the position a tight Latissimus Dorsi muscle will encourage your back to adopt (see the following chapter, **Learning Zone:** *Why* **Muscles are the Key Factor in Eliminating Your Pain***). If your back drops down too much, this will result in a position of relative lumbar extension. This is why a tight Latissimus Dorsi muscle can contribute to EDP. If you do not correct this, the exercise may end up aggravating your pain instead of easing it.*

4) FORWARD FLEXION (SITTING)

Sitting on the edge of a chair, gently lean forward as if to touch the floor (you do not have to touch the floor though, just go as far as you feel comfortable). Hold for a count of 3-5 seconds and then return to the starting position. If you find this exercise easy, progress to reaching as far back under the chair as you can.

SCHEDULE:

Repetitions: 5
Sets: 3
Times per Day: 3

5) FORWARD FLEXION (STANDING)

> *Before you progress further, it is important I highlight now the need to be careful when performing the following exercise. Although it is a movement the lower back should be more than happy to tolerate, it does nevertheless place a reasonable amount of stress across the lower back. Therefore, all I ask is for you to carry out this exercise nice and slowly and if you are in any doubt whatsoever with regard to performing this exercise, or are slightly apprehensive, continue with the previous exercise* **Forward Flexion (sitting)** *just given.*

This is similar to exercise **No 4)** only this time in standing. Gently bend forward as if to touch your toes (although like the previous exercise, you do not have to touch your toes, just go as far as you feel comfortable with). Hold for a count of 3-5 seconds and return to standing. If you feel a stretch in the back of your legs when performing this exercise, don't worry, it's no problem. However, it probably means your Hamstrings are also tight. I would therefore suggest you pay particular attention to the Hamstring stretches given on **pages 225-226** in **Step Six:** *Move Forward with Stretching Exercises.*

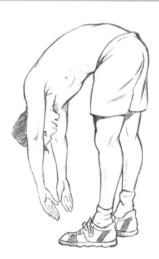

SCHEDULE:

Repetitions: 5
Sets: 3
Times per Day: 3

When performing exercises 4) and 5), make sure you tighten your stomach muscles when returning to the sitting/standing position. This will help prevent your lower back adopting an extended posture as you raise yourself up back into the upright position – see the following chapter, **Learning Zone:** *Why Muscles are the Key Factor in Eliminating Your Pain under 'How inefficiently working muscles can influence your movement' for an explanation as to why this will be beneficial.*

When performing these exercises we are looking for a decrease in pain and/or some kind of stretching in your lower/mid back, buttock or leg. The important thing to remember here is that as you perform the exercises it should *at least* feel the same from the first to the last repetition, although ideally you will find it gets easier the more repetitions you perform. This may be in the form of the pain easing, the tightness reducing or you moving further before you perceive the pain and/or tightness.

If, on the other hand, you feel that as you perform these exercises your pain increases, you need to stop. Wait for it to settle and then begin again by either taking it easier or moving back down the scale, e.g. from exercise No 3 to No 2.

If you were performing just a few light No 1 exercises **Posterior Pelvic Tilt (Lying and Standing)** and still feeling an increase in your pain, these exercises are not the ones for you *at this particular time.* Stop doing them and think about whether you are truly suffering with EDP. If you are confident you are, still give these exercises a miss for a day or two, but in the meantime, maybe try some of the resting positions given in **Step 2:** *How to STOP Acutely Inflamed Pain.* When you feel your pain has settled a little, re-introduce exercise No 1.

If, on the other hand, you feel you may have misdiagnosed your problem, still ease off on the exercises for a while, but when your pain settles, try introducing some of the exercises given earlier in this chapter for FDP.

STRETCHING AND MOVEMENT EXERCISES

The three exercises given here are what I would refer to as basic ones, and are usually the first ones for you to perform if your pain is still a little sore and irritable. These exercises can be performed regardless of what diagnosis you have given yourself, as long as they do not aggravate your pain.

1) KNEE ROLLS

Position yourself in crook lying with your knees and ankles together, then tighten your stomach muscles and gently rock your knees to one side as shown, going only as far as you feel comfortable. When you have progressed as far as you feel appropriate, gently stop and hold there for a count of 1-2 seconds and then return to the middle. Following this, gently rock your knees to the opposite side as far as you feel comfortable, and hold again for 1-2 seconds before returning to the midline. As you go to each side, ideally we are looking for a feeling of tightness/stretching around the outside of the back, hip or upper leg on the opposite side of that you are rocking to.

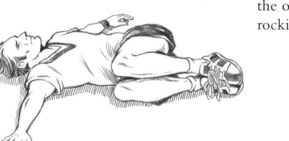

SCHEDULE:

Repetitions: 5-10 to each side
Sets: 3
Times per Day: 3

> *When performing the knee rolls exercise, be aware of any feeling you may have in the groin area of the opposite leg of the side you are rocking to. If you begin to feel any soreness or pain in this region, ease off a little, as you may be putting a little too much stress across your hip joint.*

2) THORACIC ROTATIONS

Standing as shown, turn to one side until you feel a stretch/tightness in your back. Gently 'rock' 3-4 times at the end of this range and return to the middle position. Repeat to the opposite side.

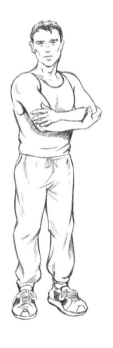

SCHEDULE:

Repetitions: 5-10 to each side
Sets: 3
Times per Day: 3

3) SIDE STRETCH

Standing in an upright position, gently side bend to one side as shown below left, until you feel a stretch on the opposite side of your back or upper leg. Gently hold for 3–5 seconds and return to the standing position.

    If you feel no stretch when performing this exercise, continue by bringing your arm 'up and over' as you side bend to the opposite side, as shown below right.

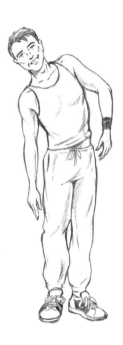

SCHEDULE:

Repetitions: 5–10 to each side
Sets: 3
Times per Day: 3

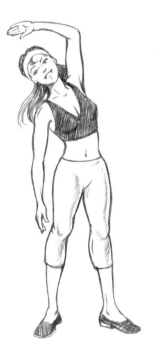

> *With all of the exercises within the Stretching and Movement Exercises section of this chapter, you are looking for a stretching sensation. If you feel no stretch at all while performing these exercises, but instead a pain that kicks in at a certain point, do not necessarily stop them. I would rather you continue the exercise but perform it within your pain-free range.*

Familiarise yourself with these exercises and perform them as you feel appropriate. When you are confident you are ready to move on to some more demanding stretching exercises, move on to the following chapter, **Learning Zone: *Why Muscles are the Key Factor in Eliminating Your Pain*** and then **Step Six: *Move Forward with Stretching Exercises.***

The former chapter explains why tight and weak muscles can lead to pain and the latter will contain a new set of advanced stretching exercises for you to perform.

Learning Zone:

Why Muscles are the Key Factor in Eliminating Your Pain

You should now be getting a good idea of how you are going to provide your body with the ideal conditions to free yourself of pain. We now need to establish the likely reason for your suffering with pain in the first place, as well as how you are going to relieve your lower back and sciatic nerve of any undue stresses. This will enable you not only to abolish your pain but actually to **DECREASE** the chances of you developing any pain again.

I really want to impress upon you the statement I have made in the last paragraph, with regard to decreasing the chances of you developing pain again.

I feel incredibly frustrated when I read books and literature which state once you have suffered with low back pain/sciatica, you will either always have that pain or always have an increased risk of developing the same pain again. *I could not disagree more.*

Providing you address the problem that was causing the pain in the first place, there is no reason why you should not be able at least to reduce, and hopefully to eliminate the chances of developing further episodes of pain. Once again, I am going to use another medical analogy here:

Let's say a middle-aged man has suffered a heart attack, primarily a result of him having a diet rich in saturated fats, smoking cigarettes and having a sedentary lifestyle. He is rushed to hospital and his life is saved.

If he were to leave hospital and change nothing with regard to his way of life, I would hazard a good guess that as time passed his chances of having a second heart attack would increase with every day. If, however, he were to take note of the warning heart attack, change his diet and general lifestyle for a healthier one and begin an appropriate exercise programme, I would equally hazard a guess that the chances of him suffering a second heart attack would decrease as time passed.

Now I'm sure you have gathered where I am going with this. The only difference between the two scenarios given above is that with the first one the individual concerned made no effort to address the underlying cause of his heart attack and consequently carried an increased risk of suffering a second one.

With the second example, however, the individual concerned looked to address the primary causes of his heart attack and therefore reduced his chances of suffering further such incidences.

So why is your back different?

The answer to this question is ***it is not!*** If you develop low back pain or sciatica and do very little about the causes of it, the chances of you encountering a second bout of pain are pretty high. I do not deny there is a reasonable chance your body will heal itself, as you will naturally avoid the aggravating factors that are causing your pain. You now know this in turn will lead to the body eventually healing itself.

However, if your pain is, like most, a result of incorrect postural or movement stresses along with muscle imbalance, these will still be present even when your body has healed itself and is pain-free. These causative factors will continue to place inappropriate stresses across your back and therefore it should come as no surprise when they eventually breach your pain threshold levels and you develop pain again.

However, if you heed the advice given and carry out the appropriate exercises in this book, you will be eliminating these undue stress factors. Consequently, you will be removing the predisposing factors for your pain and decreasing the chances of ever suffering further episodes of low back pain or sciatica again.

Therefore, even if you have been fortunate and the simple changes and exercise you have performed already have resolved your pain completely, please read through the remainder of this book and look to see if any of the given muscles are particularly tight or weak. If they are, I strongly recommend you begin to stretch and strengthen them, ***it will reduce the risk of your pain returning.***

MUSCLES, MUSCLES AND MORE MUSCLES

The remainder of this chapter will highlight how and why I believe tight and weak muscles, i.e. muscle imbalance, can predispose you to developing low back pain or sciatica. This happens due to these tight and weak muscles creating increased stresses upon your back which break through your body's pain threshold barrier. Of equal importance is not just how they can cause your initial bout of pain, but also how these same stresses can maintain your pain or put you at risk of developing further pain.

If you are unsure at all with regard to the exact whereabouts of the following muscles on your body, feel free to return the chapter, **Learning Zone:** *Your Lower Back and Sciatic Nerve to see where each muscle is positioned.*

Gluteals and Hamstrings

Both the Gluteal and Hamstring muscles have an influence over the lower back via the pelvis. I have found the main problem with these muscles tends to be tightness.

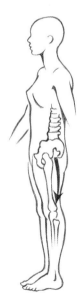

In the diagram to the right, the arrow is indicating how tight Hamstrings would pull down on the pelvis and encourage it to rotate posteriorly. As it does this, it encourages the natural lordotic curve of the lumbar spine to be flattened out, which applies a relative flexion force to the lower back. Tightness in these muscles can, in particular, aggravate the pain of someone suffering with FDP. Tight Gluteal muscles would also potentially exacerbate this problem.

A classic movement example where tight Hamstring and Gluteal muscles pose a problem would be bending forward, especially if incorrectly. As we bend forward, weight, momentum and gravity encourage the back to continue to bend, taking the pelvis along with it. However, if the Hamstrings and Gluteals are tight, they tend to resist this pull on the pelvis, because they don't have the flexibility to allow any further movement to take place. What then happens is the body takes the path of least resistance.

Therefore to gain the required movement, the body can either:

i) Pull even harder on the tight muscles, forcing them to stretch further.

ii) Take the extra movement required from the lumbar spine itself, where there are several lumbar vertebrae and a little movement from each can be gained. This is depicted in the diagram shown to the right.

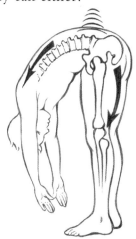

The chances are that the body will find it easier to gain a little movement from each of the vertebral segments of the lumbar spine as opposed to stretching the large, powerful tight muscles of the Gluteals and Hamstrings. This extra movement upon the lumbar vertebrae places further stresses across them, in particular the soft tissues such as muscles and ligaments, as well as the discs. If these stresses then breach the body's pain threshold level, pain will result. This scenario is typical with FDP.

In addition to this, the sciatic nerve also passes through the Hamstring muscles. Therefore, if this muscle group is tight, it will in turn place the sciatic nerve under increasing tension, potentially leading to sciatic pain, i.e. sciatica.

Piriformis

This muscle is attached to the outer part of the hip as well as the sacrum. You can see with the diagram below right, how the sciatic nerve passes in very close proximity to this muscle. It varies from person to person, but the sciatic nerve usually passes under the Piriformis muscle; however, with some people it does actually pass through it.

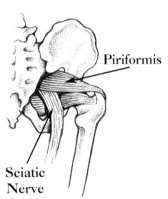

If the Piriformis muscle becomes tight or inflamed for any reason, this can aggravate the sciatic nerve. As a consequence, pain may be felt anywhere along the length of the sciatic nerve from the buttock down to the foot.

In addition to this, a tight Piriformis muscle can be responsible for a lot of low back pain due to its 'pull' on the sacrum and its potential to aggravate the Sacro-Iliac Joint.

Quadriceps and Iliopsoas

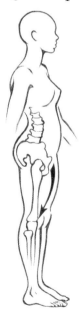

If these muscles are tight, they will also pull on the pelvis and lumbar spine. However, this time the pelvis will be pulled in the opposite direction compared to what happens if the Gluteals or Hamstrings are tight, i.e. anteriorly. The Psoas muscle is also attached to the lumbar spine itself, therefore tightness in this muscle will have the direct effect of pulling the lumbar spine into extension.

As the pelvis is pulled down by the tight Quadriceps (Rectus Femoris) and/or Iliopsoas muscles, as shown in the diagram to the left, it forces the lumbar spine into increased lordosis (relative extension), which compresses the facet joint surfaces together. This can cause these joint surfaces to be aggravated and therefore result in pain. This problem is typical with EDP.

Erector Spinae and Latissimus Dorsi

These muscles place an extension force on the lumbar spine if tight and this is often seen with those suffering with EDP.

This is due to:

Erector Spinae: these have an extension action on the lower back, therefore they tend to hold the spine in a relative state of extension if tight and unable to relax.

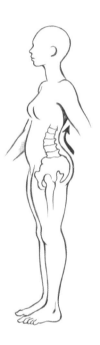

Latissimus Dorsi: this muscle will tend to pull the posterior aspect of the pelvis upwards, which in turn will create anterior tilt of the pelvis, as shown in the diagram on the right (in a similar manner to the effect a tight Quadriceps and Iliopsoas muscle can have when they pull the anterior aspect of the pelvis downwards, as previously described). This will especially be the case if your arms are placed above your head, due to this large muscle attaching to the upper part of the arm. Therefore, if this muscle is tight and you lift your arms above your head, it will pull the pelvis into anterior rotation or relative lumbar extension. This will consequently force the facet joints together again and may aggravate or lead to EDP.

The significance of this example with regard to the Latissimus Dorsi muscle, and the act of lifting your arms above your head, can be seen in activities such as back stroke when swimming. When performing this stroke, every time you take your arms up and over your head, it may 'force' your back into extension. This can potentially aggravate your pain, especially if you are suffering with EDP. (See *'Swimming is a good exercise for your bad back'* in the final chapter **Old Wives' Tales**.)

Abdominals

The problem here tends to be weakness, as the abdominal muscles play a very important role in providing stability for the lower back and pelvis. Consequently, they play an important role in holding the lumbar spine, via the pelvis, in a neutral position.

If these muscles are weak, they will find it difficult to hold up the anterior aspect of the pelvis, therefore resulting in the pelvis tipping forward (anterior rotation). This places the lumbar spine in a position of relative extension, increasing stresses upon the facet joints as found with EDP and just explained under Quadriceps and Iliopsoas, and Latissimus Dorsi.

HOW INEFFICIENTLY WORKING MUSCLES CAN INFLUENCE YOUR MOVEMENT

In addition to the examples just given, I would also like to highlight a couple of examples as to how incorrect muscular activity can result in low

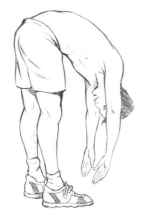

back pain/sciatica. It is not uncommon for me to see someone bend forward as if to touch their toes and as they do so there is very little movement taking place in their lower back. Nearly all the movement comes from the pelvis/hips.

As we bend forward, the natural lordotic curve of the lower back should be gradually lost as the spine begins to bend the opposite way (as seen to the left).

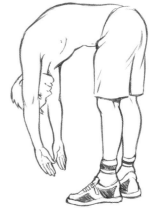

However, if the extensor muscles in the lower back, e.g. Erector Spinae, along with the other soft tissues in that region, are particularly tight, they may not 'let go' and allow the lower back to uncurl the way it should. Therefore, the back stays fairly straight and bends very little, if at all (as seen to the right on the previous page).

Under such circumstances, every time we bend forward, an increased 'stretching' stress is placed across the muscles and soft tissues of the lower back and they can become overstrained or torn. This is common with EDP. If this is the case, just like any torn soft tissue, as they heal they need to be stretched. If not, the scar tissue which results from the body's healing process will be too tight and place undue stress across the lower back again.

It is difficult for you to notice, but if someone was to observe you bending forward and they noticed your lower back stayed reasonably straight as you did so, there is a fair chance the muscles and soft tissues in your lower back are particularly tight. In addition to this, it is also possible you will feel a sensation of tightness/stretching across your lower back when bending forward.

If so, the 'flexion' stretching exercises recommended in this book for EDP will be crucial for your recovery. As always, though, be careful not to stretch too much, too soon, as this may aggravate your pain.

Moving on from this example one step further, I sometimes see patients who can bend forward and touch their toes with no pain whatsoever and the lordotic lumbar spine uncurls perfectly. Yet as they return to the standing position their pain 'kicks in'. More often than not this is a result of them over-extending their lumbar spine (increasing the lordotic curve) as they return to the standing position.

When we stand up after bending forward, our lower back should 'uncurl' as we do so, in the opposite way to which it curls forward as we bend down. If our Abdominal and Gluteal muscles are not working as well as they should, along with having over-active and/or tight Erector Spinae muscles, this can result in us over-arching (extending) our lower back as we return to the standing position.

Once again, this places increased stress upon the facet joints. If you were to over-extend like this on returning from bending forward, there is every chance you would also perform this subtly many times throughout the day, each time placing a cumulative stress across the facet joints.

This continues until eventually the pain threshold level is breached and pain is perceived. If this second example is a pattern of pain you recognise, try tightening your stomach and Gluteal muscles (clench your bottom!) before returning to the standing position; this may make it a little easier. If it does, this is an important exercise for you, as you need to encourage these muscles to work whenever you return to an upright position after bending forward.

The more you consciously work these muscles when returning to the upright position (whether while performing a specific exercise or during day-to-day activities) the more these muscles will become familiar with working while doing so. Eventually, they will naturally activate when performing such movements without you even thinking about it, therefore reducing the stress across the facet joints.

Another way potentially to recognise this type of problem, is by using your hands to 'walk up' your thighs when returning to the standing position. As you do this, imagine gently arching your back away from your stomach, i.e. moving in the opposite way to the lordotic arch your lower back naturally has. If you do this, you should find standing up is a little easier. Once again, you need to learn how to recruit the muscles about your lower back and pelvis correctly, particularly your lower Abdominals and Gluteals.

In addition to working these muscles consciously, it will also be important to strengthening your core stability muscles (**Step Seven: *Move Forward with Core Stability Exercises*)** and Gluteal muscles (***Specific Strengthening Outside Of Core Stability***) as part of a prescribed exercise programme, as well as stretching out any tight muscles which may be present in the lower back area. (See ***Treating Extension Dominated Pain*** in the previous chapter **Step Five: *Getting Moving Again.*)**

You should now have a reasonable understanding of why tight and/or weak muscles can result in pain. The following two chapters **Step Six: *Move Forward with Stretching Exercises*** and **Step Seven: *Move Forward with Core Stability Exercises*** will guide you through more challenging exercises. This will ensure your back stays supple and strong, enabling you to resolve your pain completely and also reduce the risks of you having to endure further episodes of pain.

Step Six:

Move Forward with Stretching Exercises

The following exercises will enable your back to become more mobile, therefore not only helping to eliminate the pain you have been suffering, but also significantly reducing the risks of you developing pain again.

I am going to state the obvious now, but with all of the following stretching exercises you should feel a good but comfortable stretch. The reason I am highlighting this is because the chances are you do not have tight muscles for all of the given muscles in this chapter (although I wouldn't be surprised if one or two do!). Therefore, if you carry out an exercise as described and feel no stretch at all, do not force the exercise as if you must feel a stretch. If you feel no stretch and are carrying out the exercise as described, the likelihood is the muscle concerned is not tight and therefore does not need stretching.

> *Do not forget, all exercises should be pain-free. If they are not, ease off a little or drop back to the level you know you are comfortable with. However, if you feel they are too easy, increase the intensity of the exercise or perform them more often.*

All of the stretching exercises given in this chapter should be held for approximately 20-30 seconds for each side and carried out as follows:

SCHEDULE:

Repetitions: 3 for each side
Sets: 1
Times per Day: 2-3

GLUTEAL STRETCH

Lying as shown, with your right foot positioned roughly in the region of your left knee, gently pull your right knee 'up and across' your body with your left hand. While performing this you should feel a stretch in your right buttock area. You may also feel a stretch passing down your right leg a little or into your back; as long as this is only a stretch and not painful, I do not mind. As you perform this exercise, it does not matter if your right foot lifts up and away further from your left knee. I use this description just to ensure you start the exercise in the correct position.

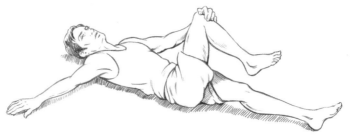

There is no magic angle across which to pull your knee. In the above example, I often say imagine drawing a line from your right to left hip and also from your right hip to your left shoulder. The angle at which you pull your knee across can be anywhere within this range. This is because the muscle being stretched is quite large and it all depends upon which part of the muscle is tightest as to the best angle to stretch it at. This particular angle may change as you progress with the exercise.

> *The warning given for Knee Rolls during* **Step 5: Getting Moving Again,** *is also relevant for this exercise, i.e. this exercise can place increased stress upon the hip joint. Therefore, if you feel any discomfort at all in the groin region, it is important to ease off a little or change the angle at which you are pulling your knee across your body.*

PIRIFORMIS STRETCH

I am going to show you three stretches for this muscle. As a rule of thumb the first one is slightly more 'gentle' than the second, which itself is slightly gentler than the third. As always, you perform the one which you feel gives you the best stretch but is also most comfortable.

N.B. Please ensure you read the following paragraphs before attempting any of the following exercises.

If, with any of the following Piriformis stretches, you find it difficult to place your ankle upon your knee as suggested, because of increased tightness or pain, straighten the knee upon which your ankle is resting. Having done this, you should find it a little easier to place your ankle upon it. If need be, you can have the knee of the appropriate leg completely straight or maybe place your ankle somewhere along your shin as opposed to on your knee.

If you do take this approach, when you feel a stretch, continue with the exercise in this new position. As the exercise becomes easier, begin to slide your ankle further up your shin towards your knee and/or bend your knee further towards the original position given, whichever is appropriate.

Although this stretch is targeting the Piriformis muscle, and therefore the aim is to feel the stretch in and around the buttock area, people sometimes state they feel a stretch around the front of their groin. Without doubt, this is not stretching the Piriformis muscle. However, the likelihood is that it's stretching tight soft tissues about the front of your groin, and it is these tight tissues that are preventing you from stretching far enough to address the Piriformis muscle.

As long as it is *only* stretching/tightness you are feeling, continue with the stretch. As you do so, the soft tissues at the front of you groin should become more supple and will therefore allow you to address the Piriformis muscle. You will know when this is happening due to the stretching now being felt more towards the buttock region.

If you did notice a stretching more in the groin area as opposed to the buttock, I would pay particular attention to the Quadriceps, Iliopsoas and Adductor stretches given later in this chapter, as these muscles may also be tight.

If you are finding it difficult to perform this exercise, the reason is likely to be due to your Piriformis muscle being extremely tight. This is relatively common and as I have alluded to before, tightness with this muscle is probably one of the most common individual causes of low back pain and sciatica I find. Therefore, although I want you to be careful, it is even more reason to persevere with this exercise, as it may be one of the main reasons you are suffering with pain in the first place.

i)   Lying as shown, place your left ankle upon your right knee and your left hand upon your left knee. Gently push your left knee away from you with your left hand until you feel a stretching sensation in your left buttock region, although, as with the Gluteal stretch, you may find this stretch creeps down the leg or up into the back.

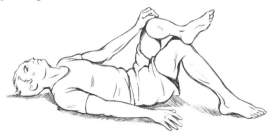

ii) If you feel no stretch at all with the previous exercise, progress by pulling your right knee gently towards your chest with your right hand, while still maintaining a gentle pressure against your left knee, as shown.

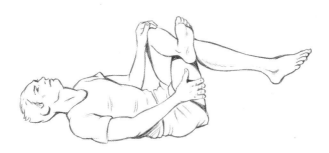

Once again, we are looking for a similar stretch to that previously described. An alternative to this can be performed by holding behind your left ankle with your right hand and then pulling your ankle towards your chest instead of your right knee. Either way, the aim is to take your left knee and ankle closer to your chest.

iii) If you feel no stretch with the previous two Piriformis exercises, or you feel you would like to increase the stretch you are feeling, carry out a similar exercise in sitting. Sitting on the edge of a chair, rest your left ankle upon your right knee while keeping your back relaxed but straight, as shown to the right. If you feel a stretch already, hold this position as this is your stretch. To progress, however, gently push down on your left knee until you feel the appropriate stretch. If you still feel nothing, gently lean forward at the hips while keeping your back straight.

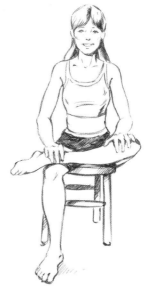

You should feel a stretching sensation around your left buttock area, although as described with the first stretch, this may also be felt towards the back or down the leg slightly.

Remember, as I mentioned at the beginning of these Piriformis stretches, if you feel it is too difficult to perform any of these exercises, try straightening the knee a little of the side *not being stretched* or slide the heel of the side that is being stretched a little further below your knee/down your shin.

Self Massage

Some people find it beneficial to massage a tight Piriformis muscle themselves in order to loosen it up a little. One of the best ways to do this is to find a small firm ball, maybe a tennis ball or something a little smaller (some people like using a golf ball, although this can be a little too firm) and then place yourself in the crook lying position.

While in this position, place the ball under the middle of the buttock area on the side where the Piriformis muscle is tight. Be careful, but then simply massage this area by increasing and decreasing the weight going through the ball as well as moving the ball gently in circles.

Perform this for a few minutes, maybe twice a day.

---

*It is important to proceed with caution with this self-massaging exercise, as this muscle can be extremely tender and also the sciatic nerve passes in the same vicinity. Nevertheless, if this muscle is tight and knotted, it can also be an excellent way to make it more supple. The usual rules apply…**listen to your body,** as this exercise should not aggravate your signs and symptoms. This area may feel a little bruised after performing this exercise. If this is the case but you feel your pain is easing, proceed with caution. However, be careful not to aggravate your signs and symptoms.*

HAMSTRING STRETCH

There are many different ways to stretch the Hamstring muscles and I am giving you three of my 'favourites'. The intensity of stretch given should increase as you progress through each of the three exercises. Feel free to try others, as long as they do not reproduce your pain and give a similar stretch to that described:

i) Lying as shown and holding behind one knee, gently tighten your stomach muscles as you gently straighten the knee you are holding. You should feel a stretch in the back of this leg.

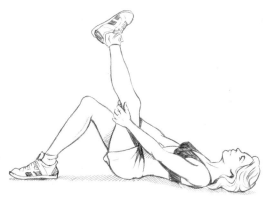

ii) Sitting on the edge of a chair as shown, with your back straight and right leg slightly bent but out in front of you,

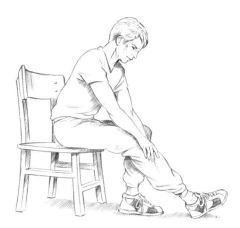

gently lean forward at your hips until you feel a stretch down the back of your leg. If you lean as far forward as you can and yet you still feel no stretch, then staying bent forward at the hips gently straighten your right knee further.

iii) If you feel you want to be a little more aggressive with your Hamstring stretch, sit on the floor as shown with your left knee bent and out to the side and your right knee slightly bent but out in front of you. Keeping your back straight, gently lean forward at your hips until you feel a stretch down the back of your right leg. If you feel no stretch while doing this, after bending forward at the hips, gently straighten your right leg until you feel a stretch down the back of it.

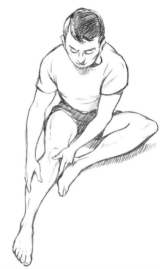

As you will now be aware, the Hamstring muscle travels from the pelvis to attach just below the knee. When performing these exercises, it is not unusual to feel the stretch pass below the knee and into the calf muscle. As the Hamstring muscle does not pass into the calf, the stretch you are feeling cannot be due to this muscle, but rather the nervous system, and in particular the sciatic nerve and its branches. However, if the nervous system is tight it still needs stretching, so please continue with this exercise as described, as long as it is only a stretch/tightness you are feeling and not pain.

If you do feel a stretch in the calf area as mentioned, be sure to try the calf stretches given later in this chapter. Although this does not indicate tight calf muscles as such, if the nervous system is a little tight, it is best to stretch all potential tight interfaces, and the calf muscles may be one of them.

Another thing I wish to note here is that as you are performing this stretch, it is not uncommon to feel pins and needles in your foot/lower leg. If you do notice this, I am not too concerned as long as it resolves itself within a few minutes of stretching (and obviously that it is not generally worsening any of your signs and symptoms). Once again, this can occur due to the sciatic nerve passing through the Hamstring muscles.

If you are carrying out this stretch with a bias towards the sciatic nerve, the nerve itself may not function 100 per cent as it is being stretched, sometimes resulting in sensations such as pins and needles. As I stated above, as long as this resolves itself within a few minutes of stopping and standing up, I am not too concerned. It should not, however, hang around for much longer than this or generally worsen any of you signs and symptoms. If it does, ease off on this stretch or stop it altogether for a while until your signs and symptoms improve.

QUADRICEPS STRETCH

I have provided three stretches for the Quadriceps muscle. You will read that Hamstring cramps can sometimes be a problem with this exercise, therefore the second and third exercises here are just a modification of the first exercise to try and prevent any problems you may encounter.

> ### *Beware of Hamstring cramps!*
> *This can be difficult to address and typically occurs when you have tight Hamstring muscles as well. To try and address this, first you need to make sure your Hamstring muscles are as relaxed as possible when performing this exercise.*
> *Therefore, you may find stretching your Hamstring muscles before performing this exercise helps.*
> *Your Hamstring muscles are used to bend your knee up to place your foot towards your buttock. What tends to happen here is that the Hamstring muscles become overused in their shortened position as you actively bring your foot up towards your buttock, instead of relaxing the muscle and using only your hand to pull your foot up. Therefore, one way to try and prevent this is to relax the Hamstrings as much as possible and make sure it is your hand that lifts your foot up.*

i) Standing as shown, keeping your back straight and gently tightening your stomach muscles, take hold of your left ankle and gently pull it up towards your left buttock. You should feel a stretch around the front of your thigh.

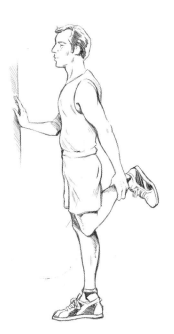

If you are finding this exercise quite difficult, due to Hamstring cramps or any other reason, the following alternatives may help:

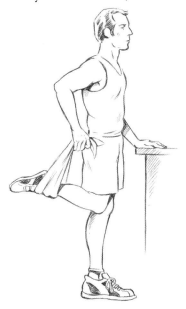

ii) If this muscle is particularly tight and you find it difficult to grasp your ankle, you may wish to use a towel to assist. Place the towel around your ankle and use the ends of the towel to pull your foot up towards your buttock.

iii) Another way to try and prevent any problems is to carry out the exercise in side lying. The stretch is performed exactly the same as described with the previous exercise, either with or without the towel, but modified by lying on the opposite side of the leg you wish to stretch.

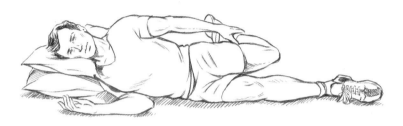

Be aware of some incorrect movements which can occur when performing the Quadriceps stretch:

➤ *Keep your knees together.* Some people have a tendency to pull their leg away from the mid-line when performing this exercise. It is best to keep your knees fairly close to each other.

➤ *Keep your back straight* This is vitally important. If you need to perform this stretch there is a reasonable chance, but not definite, you are suffering with EDP. When performing this exercise, there can be a tendency for people to over-arch their back (extension). If you were to do this, it may begin to aggravate your pain. Make sure you are tightening your stomach muscles, as this will help to keep your back straight.

➤ *Leaning Forward* Although this will probably not aggravate your pain, it is unnecessary. Some people tend to keep their back straight but then lean forwards at the hips as they carry out this exercise, i.e. they end up looking towards the floor. As I mentioned, it is unlikely to aggravate your pain by doing this but it is not the correct way to perform this exercise.

ILIOPSOAS STRETCH

The following are two stretches for the Iliopsoas muscle. They are both very similar so choose whichever one you find gives you the best stretch.

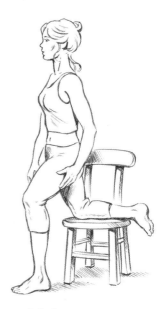

i) Standing as shown, with the knee of the side to be stretched resting on a chair and the other leg a small stride in front, gently tighten your stomach muscles as you bend your stance leg as if to lunge forward. As you lunge forward, it is important not to over-arch/extend your back. Imagine you are simply pushing your pelvis forward while keeping your back straight. The aim is to feel a stretch in the front of your hip/groin region of the leg resting on the chair, although if your Quadriceps are particularly tight, you may feel the stretch passing down the front of your thigh as well.

If you are not feeling much of a stretch, be careful, but try stepping forward a little further with your stance leg.

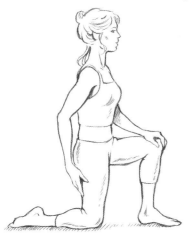

ii) Placing yourself on the floor as shown, with the knee of the side to be stretched on the floor and the opposite leg out in front of you, gently 'lunge' or 'push' the knee of the front leg forward. While doing this, it is important you keep your back straight as described in the previous Iliopsoas stretch. You should feel a stretch in the groin region.

However, if the Quadriceps are particularly tight, you may feel a stretch down the front of your thigh as previously mentioned.

> *As with the Quadriceps stretch, sometimes people tend to over arch their back (extension) when performing these stretches. This could aggravate your pain, especially if your diagnosis is EDP. This is why it is vitally important to keep the back straight and tighten your stomach muscles while performing this exercise.*

LATISSIMUS DORSI STRETCH

This stretch is pretty much the same as the four-point kneeling flexion exercise given in **Step Five:** *Getting Moving Again.* Placing yourself on all fours, with your hands approximately underneath your shoulders and knees below your hips, keep your hands in the same position and gently arch your back up toward the ceiling (only as far as you feel appropriate) and then lean backwards as if to sit on your heels as shown. We are looking for a stretch around your lower back area.

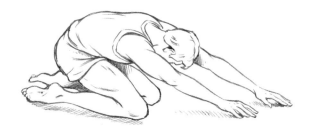

However, you may also feel a stretch further up your back towards your shoulders. If you feel no stretch at all while performing this exercise, keeping your bottom close to your heels, gently stretch your hands further in front of you. Once again we are looking for a stretch in the similar areas.

If your buttock muscles (Gluteals) are particularly tight, you may also feel a stretch in the buttock region, as long as it is only a stretch then this is no problem. However, I would suggest you try the Gluteal stretch given earlier in this chapter as well.

*It is important when performing this exercise to keep the back arched upwards, even if only a little. There can be a tendency to allow your back to 'drop down' when performing this exercise. This is exactly the position a tight Latissimus Dorsi muscle will encourage your back to adopt. For more on this see the previous chapter, **Learning Zone: Why Muscles are the Key Factor in Eliminating Your Pain.** If your back drops down too much, this will result in a position of relative lumbar extension. This is why a tight Latissimus Dorsi muscle can contribute to EDP. If you do not correct this, this exercise may end up aggravating your pain instead of easing it.*

ADDUCTOR STRETCHES

There are two possible stretches for the Adductor muscles, which are positioned on the inner part of your thigh.

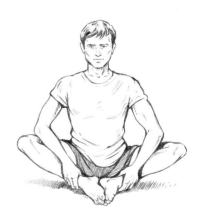

i)   Sitting with the soles of your feet facing each other as shown, place your elbows/forearms on the inside of your knees and then gently 'push' your knees outwards until you feel a stretch on the inner part of each thigh. If you can only feel it on one thigh, this simply indicates that one side is tighter than the other.

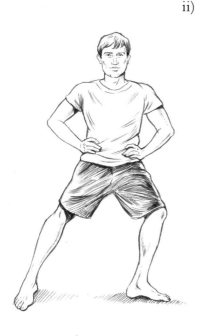

ii)   Standing as shown, with the foot of your right leg pointing in front of you and the foot and knee of your bent left leg pointing to the side, gently tighten your stomach muscles and bend your left leg further as if you are lunging to the left side, while all the time continuing to look and keep your body facing forwards. You should begin to feel a stretch on the inner part of your right thigh. Change over legs and repeat for the other side.

GASTROCNEMIUS STRETCH

The Gastrocnemius muscle is the bigger of the two muscles often referred to as the calf muscles. This muscle is attached just above the knee joint and passes down to the heel. This is why the knee must be kept straight when performing this exercise.

To perform this stretch, stand facing a wall as shown to the right, with your feet approximately hip width apart and your right leg behind your left. Gently lean towards the wall while ensuring your heels remain on the floor, your toes point forward and your right knee is straight. If this muscle is tight, you should feel a stretch at the back of your right leg, anywhere from the back of your knee to the just above your ankle.

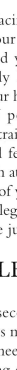
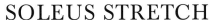

SOLEUS STRETCH

The second of the calf muscles is the smaller Soleus muscle, this muscle does not pass across the knee but rather attaches just below it before passing down the leg. It is for this reason that the knee is bent while stretching this muscle.

To perform this stretch, stand facing a wall as shown to the left, with your feet approximately hip width apart. However, as opposed to having your right leg behind your

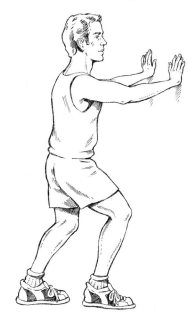

235

left and keeping your knee straight, as is done with the Gastrocnemius stretch, this time place your right leg in front of your left leg and keep your knee bent.

While in this position, gently 'push' your right knee towards the wall while ensuring your right heel remains on the floor and your toes are pointing forward. If this muscle is tight, you should feel a stretch at the back of your leg, anywhere from just below your knee to just above your ankle.

All of the exercises in the chapter have shown you how to stretch any tight muscles that may be contributing to your pain. Work out the ones that you feel are tight and then incorporate them into a gentle stretching exercise programme.

The following chapter **Step Seven: *Move Forward with Core Stability Exercises*** will show you how to strengthen the important stabilising muscles for your lower back and pelvis.

Step Seven:

Move Forward with Core Stability Exercises

There seems to be a trend of late with regard to 'core stability', i.e. working specific muscles that help stabilise the lower back and pelvis. In particular there has been an emphasis on the Transversus Abdominis (TA) and Multifidus muscles. Before I progress any further with this chapter, I would just like to share my thoughts with regard to this concept.

I am all for working any muscles which help stabilise the lower back and pelvis, I feel it is an integral part of any rehabilitation programme. However, there appears to be an emphasis on isolating certain muscles in order for your back to gain 'core stability' and it is this concept I do not necessarily agree with.

With these exercises, the emphasis is usually on the TA and Multifidus muscles. My problem with this is that these muscles do not work in isolation when we go about our day-to-day activities, so why try to train them in this way? That's even assuming you can!

My concept of core stability exercises refers to working the muscles which help to maintain the lower back and pelvis in a good neutral position, without too much conscious effort, i.e. not over-compensating by using incorrect muscles to 'hold' your back in a neutral position. Therefore, if you can perform a specific exercise in a nice, relaxed and controlled manner (without holding your breath) and you are also able to maintain a neutral spine while doing so, you will be working your core stability muscles.

Personally, I have found these exercises to be more appropriate, although not exclusively, for those patients suffering with EDP. This is usually because when the lower back and pelvis lack stability, the pelvis tends to rotate anteriorly and places the lower back in a position of relative extension. If this continues to happen, EDP can result. However, that is not to say only those suffering with EDP should perform these strengthening exercises, the more stability your lower back and pelvis have the better, regardless of your diagnosis.

Some of the exercises in this chapter are often described elsewhere as being for either the TA or Multifidus muscles. I would just like to highlight the fact I do not necessarily think exercises that are said to isolate these muscles are inappropriate; rather, I am not convinced they actually do isolate that particular muscle. Instead, they work all of the muscles that contribute to lower-back stability.

Like all muscles in the body, if you place appropriate increased stresses across the core stability muscles, they will respond to this by increasing their strength in order to cope with this increased stress. The following exercises aim to gradually increase the stresses across the stabilising muscles of your lower back, so they can respond to this by becoming stronger and stronger.

LOWER BACK STABILITY EXERCISES

The following exercises in this chapter do not necessarily have to be carried out in the order given. If you wish to try one specific group before another, e.g. the multifidus-biased exercises before the abdominal-biased ones, then feel free to do so. I would probably recommend you see which group you find most comfortable and begin with those. As long as you can perform them relaxed and pain-free, while maintaining a neutral posture and not holding your breath, I do not mind.

If, while performing any of the abdominal-biased exercises, you begin to aggravate your pain and/or find it difficult to maintain a neutral lumbar spine, the position just prior to that becomes your stopping point. Even if your leg has not fully straightened (exercises 1, 2, & 5) or your hip and knee are not at 90 degrees (exercises 3 & 4) it does not matter. Return to the starting position and continue the exercise with the opposite leg, but only to as far as you progressed with the first leg. For more on this see the chapter, **Learning Zone:** *The Principles of Exercise* with regard to finding any exercises easier on one side compared to the other.

You may also hear or feel a clunking noise while performing these exercises. The chances are this is coming from your hip. Although this is not harmful in any way, it still shows a decrease in stability for that region and should therefore be avoided. If this happens, do not stop the exercise completely; rather, only straighten your leg as far as you can without any 'clunking' noise.

As you continue with these exercises on a daily basis, you will find you can eventually perform the given exercise while maintaining a pain-free, neutral spine; it will then be time to progress to the next level.

THE 'NEUTRAL SPINE' POSITION

The first two exercises given in this chapter begin with you in the crook lying position. It is important that when you start these exercises, the spine is in its 'neutral spine' position. (See the chapter, **Learning Zone:** *Your Lower Back and Sciatic Nerve.*) Probably the simplest way to achieve this is to lie in the crook lying position as shown below.

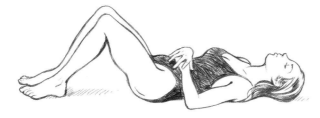

Once you are comfortably in this position, gently 'flatten' your lower back into the floor. When you have done this, gently perform the opposite movement, whereby you arch your back away from the floor. Perform this movement gently 2–3 times and then finally 'relax' your back into the mid position between the two. Your back should now be approximately in the neutral spine position.

N.B. Take care when performing this action to obtain a neutral spine, as when you are flattening your lower back into the floor, or arching it away from the floor, you could aggravate your pain whether you are suffering with either FDP or EDP. Always perform these movements only as far as you can pain-free.

ABDOMINAL BIASED EXERCISES

The following five exercises, although generally working all of the stabilising muscles of the lower back, tend to bias the abdominal muscles. They should be carried out as follows, unless stated otherwise:

SCHEDULE:

Repetitions: 5 – 10 times for each side
Sets: 3
Times per Day: 2 – 3

Taking a rest while exercising

When performing the following exercises, especially for the first time, it is likely you may find even five repetitions too much for your lower back without having to have some kind of rest – no problem. What I usually suggest, to start with, is that as soon as you have straightened your leg (exercises 1, 2 & 5) or bent your hip & knee (exercises 3 & 4) on one side as far as is appropriate, return to the crook lying resting position. Have a quick relax and then re-tighten your abdominal muscles before repeating the same exercise with the opposite leg. Once again, when you have completed the appropriate movement with that leg, return to the crook lying position, relax and re-tighten your abdominal muscles and repeat again with the leg you first used.

As you continue with the exercises, you will find you do not necessarily need to have a rest after exercising each leg…no problem, do not have a rest then. What I am saying is: do not feel you have to perform all the repetitions without a quick relax and re-tightening of your abdominals in-between, feel free to if you wish.

However, the more repetitions you can do without resting, the stronger your lower back will become, as long as you can do so while maintaining a pain-free, neutral spine.

1) Leg Slides with full support

Starting in the crook lying position, with your lower back in its neutral position as described before, gently tighten your abdominal muscles and then slide the foot of one leg along the floor as if to straighten it (as shown below).

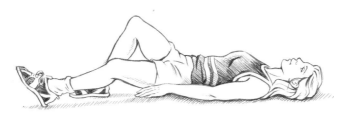

If at any stage as you are straightening your leg, you feel any pain or cannot maintain a neutral spine (without over-tensing your muscles or holding your breath) that becomes your stopping point and you should then return to the starting 'crook lying' position. Then relax and re-tighten your abdominal muscles and repeat the same process with your opposite leg.

2) Leg Slides without touching the floor

When you find the previous exercise easy, I would ask you to perform this similar, but slightly more difficult exercise. As with exercise 1), you start in the crook lying position. However, rather than sliding your leg along the floor, I am going to ask you to ensure your leg is an inch or two **above the floor** as you straighten it.

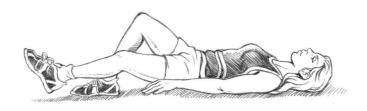

By not allowing the floor to help support your leg, it means you are asking for a little more support from your lower back. As long as your back can provide this while maintaining a pain-free neutral spine, it is no problem. The extra support being demanded from your back will help strengthen it.

The following two exercises could be said to be preparatory ones for **Leg Slides with no support,** exercise 5) on the opposite page.

3) Single Knee Raise

Starting in the crook lying position, gently tighten your abdominal muscles and raise one leg into the air, so your hip and knee are at approximately 90 degrees (as shown to the right). Hold this position for a count of 5-10 and then return to the crook lying position.

Relax and repeat for the opposite leg.

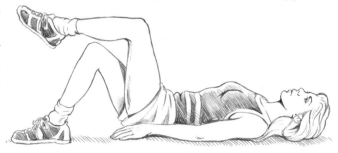

4) Double Knee Raise

Starting in the crook lying position again, gently tighten your abdominal muscles and then raise one leg into the same position as with the previous exercise. When this leg is in the correct position, follow with the other leg until you are lying with both hips and knees at 90 degrees, as shown to the left.

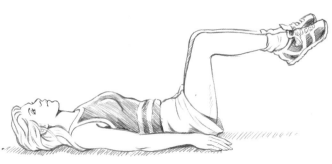

Hold this position for a count of 5-10 and then return to the crook lying position, one leg at a time.

The schedule for this last exercise is slightly different, simply because the exercise is working both legs and not each one separately. Therefore, the schedule is as follows:

SCHEDULE:

Repetitions: 5 – 10
Sets: 3
Times per Day: 2 – 3

N.B. When performing this last exercise, alternate the leg with which you lead each time, both when raising them in the air and lowering them again. For example, the first time you may wish to lead with your right, followed by your left when raising and lowering your legs. If so, I would then suggest for the next repetition you lead with your left leg first followed by your right. Continue to alternate like this until you have completed the exercise.

5) Leg Slides with no support

This is a continuation of the previous 'Leg Slides' exercises 1) and 2), only we are going to be decreasing the base of support further by not allowing either of your feet to touch the floor. Once again, this will demand more support from your lower back. Providing you can perform this exercise with a pain-free neutral spine though, the extra support demanded from your back will help strengthen it.

We are going to start in the 'Double Knee Raise' position given with Exercise 4). However, once you are in this position, I am going to ask you to slide one leg gently out in front of you with it remaining about an inch or two above the floor, just as you did with Exercise 2), *Leg Slides without touching the floor.*

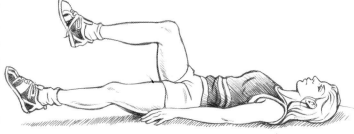

When you have straightened this

leg as far as you can while maintaining a neutral, pain-free spine, return to the starting position. Relax, re-tighten your abdominals and repeat with the opposite leg.

> *Remember, if you cannot perform any of the previous exercises without feeling pain, losing the neutral spine position or feeling a 'clunk' from your hip, then the position of your leg just prior to that is your stopping point. Continue with that exercise, taking your leg only to this point. You will find with time you can progress further.*

MULTIFIDUS-BIASED EXERCISES

The following group of six exercises will be biasing the muscles in the posterior aspect of your back a little more, and are sometimes given as exercises for the Multifidus muscle. However, they still require good abdominal strength and stability. Therefore, keeping an eye on a neutral posture is, as always, crucial.

These exercises can be divided into two groups:

➤ Those performed in prone lying: Exercises 1) – 3)
➤ Those performed in four-point kneeling: Exercises 4) – 6)

I would suggest you perform these exercises in the logical sequence of 1) to 2) to 3), etc., progressing from one to the next as one exercise becomes easy to perform.

You may at some stage, while performing these exercises, find you have:

i) Aggravated your pain.
ii) Found it difficult to maintain a neutral lumbar spine.
iii) Begun to 'wobble' about or feel unstable. (This only really applies to exercises 4) – 6) in four point kneeling.)

If so, stop performing that particular exercise and either keep to that number of repetitions or, if you were only performing one or two, drop back to the previous level.

As you progress with the exercises on a daily basis, you will find you become more adept at performing them and begin to find them quite easy. When you do, it will be time to move on to the next exercise.

The following six exercises should be carried out as follows:

SCHEDULE:

Repetitions: 5-10 times for each side
Sets: 3
Times per Day: 2 – 3

1) Prone Arm Raise

Lying prone, ensuring your back is in its neutral position, gently tighten your stomach muscles and raise one arm approximately 6 inches or so in the air. As soon as you have raised this arm, hold for a brief count of 3 and then slowly lower. Repeat for the opposite arm.

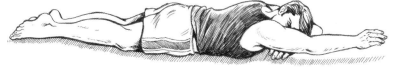

2) Prone Leg Raise

Lying prone, ensuring your back is in its neutral position, gently tighten your stomach muscles and, keeping your knee straight, raise one leg approximately 6 inches or so in the air. As soon as you have raised this leg, hold for a brief count of 3 and then slowly lower. Repeat for the opposite leg.

3) Prone 'cross-overs'

This combines the previous two exercises. Lying prone, ensuring your back is in its neutral position, gently tighten your stomach muscles and raise one leg and the opposite arm as shown, approximately 6 inches or so in the air. As soon as you have raised them, hold for a brief count of 3 and then slowly lower. Repeat again with the opposite sides.

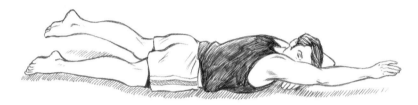

4) Four Point Kneeling Arm Raise

Kneeling on all fours, ensuring your back is in its neutral position, gently raise up one arm as if to straighten it out in front of you as shown. Hold there for a brief count of 3 and then return to all fours. Repeat again with the opposite arm.

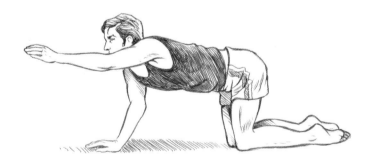

5) Four Point Kneeling Leg Raise

Kneeling on all fours and ensuring your back is in its neutral position, gently raise up one leg as if to straighten it out behind you as shown. Hold there for a brief count of 3 and then return to all fours. Repeat with the opposite leg.

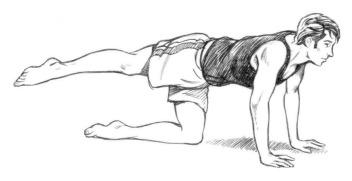

6) Four Point Kneeling 'cross-overs'

This combines the previous two exercises. Kneeling on all fours, ensuring your back is in its neutral position, raise one leg and the opposite arm together as shown. Hold for a brief count of 3 and then return to all fours. Repeat with the opposite sides.

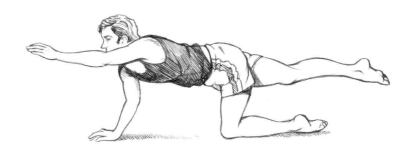

Remember, if you cannot straighten either arm and/or leg fully without feeling pain, losing the neutral spine position or feeling particularly unstable, the position of your arm and/or leg prior to that is your stopping point. Continue with the exercise taking your arm and/or leg only to this point. You will find with time you can progress further.

'GLOBAL' CORE STABILITY EXERCISES

The following two exercises place the emphasis on working the whole of the 'Global' stabilising system and not biasing certain parts of it.

Once again these will work the stabilising muscles of your lower back as you aim to maintain your neutral spine while performing them. There can be a tendency to over-arch (extend) your lower back while performing these exercises, so be careful (especially if you are suffering with EDP).

When performing the following exercises, only lift your bottom to the maximum of it being in line with your chest and thighs.

SCHEDULE:

Repetitions: 5 – 10 times
Sets: 3
Times per Day: 2 – 3

1) Bridging

Begin in the crook lying position, as described earlier in this chapter, and then gently tighten your stomach muscles and raise your bottom so it is clear of the surface you are lying on, as shown.

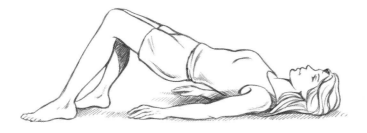

Hold this position for a count of 5-10 seconds and then relax. As you find this easy, gradually lift your bottom further from the surface you are lying on, always ensuring your pelvis stays in the neutral position and that your body is steady and not wobbling around.

2) Single Leg Bridging

This is similar to the bridging exercise just given, only this time after having tightened your stomach muscles and lifted your bottom from the floor, gently lift one leg from the floor as shown. Hold for 5-10 seconds and return to the crook lying position. Follow this by repeating the same with your other leg.

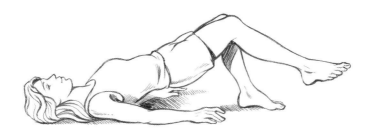

As with the first bridging exercise, if you find this easy, gradually lift your bottom further from the surface you are lying on before raising one foot from the floor, always ensuring your pelvis stays in the neutral position and that your body is steady and not wobbling around.

N.B. If you feel your Hamstrings beginning to 'overwork' with either of the previous two exercises, either consciously tighten your Gluteal and abdominal muscles a little more or lower yourself down and rest. This can happen as a result of the Hamstrings compensating for weak Gluteal muscles, and if you are not careful, your Hamstring muscles may 'cramp up'.

The important factor to remember when performing these last two exercises, is that once again the lower back and pelvis should maintain a neutral position at all times. In particular with the last one, where you are only using one leg to hold your pelvis from the floor, there can be a tendency for one side to deviate or drop down to the side. If this happens just prior to this is your stopping point. It is important only to take the exercise as far as you can without any asymmetry.

This chapter, **Step Seven: *Move Forward with Core Stability Exercises***, is without doubt integral with regard to resolving your low back pain or sciatica, as the core stability muscles play a crucial role in the functioning of your lower back and pelvis. However, the following chapter ***Specific Strengthening Outside of Core Stability*** will show you how to strengthen other muscles that may be contributing to your pain. This will continue to reduce any inappropriate stress across your lower back and sciatic nerve, therefore further encouraging healing to take place.

I have included this chapter as an additional one as it consists of exercises that I do not tend to prescribe a great deal. Nevertheless, I am not going to be complacent, as I do prescribe them from time to time and therefore have introduced them at the end of the main exercising chapters.

Specific Strengthening Outside of Core Stability

With the following exercises, it can be difficult to say whether any muscle group is particularly weak. The reason for this is that when a muscle is working to provide stability, it is different to when it is being asked to provide power and strength. More specific control is needed with stability, whereas quick powerful movements can sometimes disguise underlying instability.

With this in mind, I'm sure you will not be too surprised to hear me say, *"Listen to your body."* If you carry out some of the following exercises and feel you are not benefiting from them, the chances are you are not. Therefore, you do not need to perform them. The opposite is obviously true, in that if you perform one of the following exercises and can 'really feel it working' or maybe just find it quite challenging to perform, the chances are you need to work and strengthen that particular muscle group, therefore continue with it.

This may sound like I'm sitting on the fence once again but it's one of the many expressions I have used throughout this book, ones I hear all the time from patients. For example, patients often remark that a certain exercise '*feels really good*' or '*feels like it's making my back stronger*'. To these people I would simply say continue with that exercise and progress as you feel appropriate. I also have some patients state they tried a specific exercise but '*it didn't feel like it was doing anything*' or '*it wasn't making any difference*'. As long as they had tried the exercises and made them more challenging as appropriate, I would probably say it is okay to stop performing them and encourage them to try a different type of exercise.

Truth be told, I do not tend to give these exercises out a great deal. This is because I do not tend to find that weakness in these muscle groups contributes to low back pain and sciatica much. Nevertheless, without doubt, they can contribute to pain and there are occasions when I do use them: therefore I have included them within this book in case you are one of the individuals who may find them beneficial.

Some people may say that it can take weeks for any benefit to be recognised from specific exercises. While I agree to a certain extent, I have found this tends to be more a case of the 'uninjured' individual who is looking simply to get stronger.

However, my experience tells me that when there are muscle groups which are significantly underperforming and therefore contributing towards dysfunction and subsequent pain, the benefits tend to be noticed much quicker than this. This is why I say if no improvement is noticed within a couple of weeks, something needs to be changed.

It is important I stress here that I am not saying there will be 100 per cent improvement within this time, although sometimes there can be. Rather you should notice some kind of improvement, be it your levels of pain are reducing, you are gaining more mobility or quite simply the exercises are becoming easier to perform. Either way, it is likely to be due to the muscles becoming stronger and/or more efficient at performing their task. This in turn will help resolve your pain.

Feel free to try the following exercises with a similar principle in mind and perform them as you feel appropriate. By doing this, you will gain benefit by ridding yourself of your pain and also preventing any further episodes of pain. Remember, listen to and work with your body, it will without doubt help guide you through the exercises that are best for you.

If you are unsure as to the exact whereabouts and actions of the given muscles, just return to the chapter, **Learning Zone: *Your Lower Back and Sciatic Nerve*** where all is explained.

Finally, there is a large overlap with all of the following exercises. By this, I mean none of the exercises work exclusively the specific muscles I have highlighted; they also work other muscles. For example, you will see the bridging exercise is given for both the Gluteal and the Hamstring muscles. All of the following exercises are pretty much interchangeable, as they all give the Gluteals, Hamstrings and Quadriceps a good workout.

The schedule for each given exercise is placed at the end of each exercise/ group of exercises.

GLUTEAL EXERCISES

1) Bridging

Beginning in the crook lying position, gently tighten your stomach muscles and raise your bottom so it is clear of the surface you are lying on as shown below. Hold this position for a count of 5-10 seconds and relax. As you find this easy, gradually lift your bottom further from the surface you are lying on, always ensuring your pelvis stays in the neutral position and you do not over-extend your lower back while doing so, especially if you are suffering with EDP. It is also important your body is steady and not wobbling around.

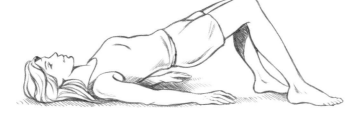

2) Single Leg Bridging

This is similar to the previous bridging exercise, only this time after having tightened your stomach muscles and lifted your bottom from the floor, gently lift one leg from the floor as shown. Hold for 5-10 seconds and return to the crook lying position. Follow this by repeating with your other leg.

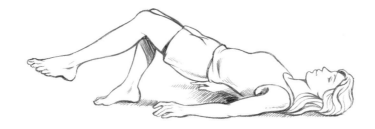

As with the first bridging exercise, if you find this easy, gradually lift your bottom further from the surface you are lying on before raising one foot from the floor, always ensuring your pelvis stays in the neutral position and that your body is steady and not wobbling around.

3) Bridging on a chair

This exercise is similar to the first bridging exercise given on the previous page, only instead of your feet resting on the floor, have them resting on a small stool/chair. As always, ensure you maintain a neutral spine.

With your feet resting upon the stool/chair, gently tighten your stomach muscles and raise your bottom so it is clear of the surface you are lying on (as shown). Hold this position for a count of 5-10 seconds and relax. As you find this easy, gradually lift your bottom further from the surface you are lying on, always ensuring your pelvis stays in the neutral position and you do not over-extend your lower back while doing so, especially if you are suffering with EDP. It is also important your body is steady and not wobbling around.

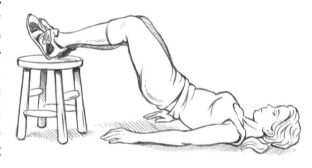

Schedule:

Repetitions: 5 –10 times
Sets: 3
Times per Day: 2 – 3

N.B. If you feel your Hamstrings begin to 'overwork' with any of the previous three exercises, either consciously tighten your Gluteal and Abdominal muscles a little more or lower yourself down and rest. This can happen as a result of the Hamstrings compensating for weak Gluteal muscles, and, if you are not careful, your Hamstring muscles may 'cramp up'.

The important factor to remember when performing the previous three bridging exercises is that once again the lower back and pelvis should maintain a neutral position at all times. In particular with 'single leg bridging' where you are only using one leg to hold your pelvis from the floor, there can be a tendency for one side to deviate or drop down to the side. If this happens, just prior to this is your stopping point. It is important to only take the exercise as far as you can without any asymmetry.

Also, never lift your bottom any higher than it being in line with your chest and thighs.

4) Small Knee Bends

Standing against a wall as shown, gently tighten your stomach and buttock muscles and then slide down the wall. While performing this exercise ensure your hips, knees and second toe are approximately in line with each other and that your hip and knees only bend to a **maximum** of 60 degrees.

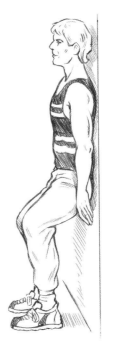

When you have lowered yourself to an appropriate level, only hold for a count of 1 or 2 and then slowly raise yourself up again. All the time ensuring you are consciously tightening your stomach and Gluteal muscles.

SCHEDULE:

Repetitions: 5 – 10 times
Sets: 3
Times per Day: 2 – 3

5) Lunges

While standing, gently tighten your stomach muscles and keep your back straight. Step forward with your right leg as if to start walking. As your foot is about to touch the floor, tighten your right buttock muscle until your foot is flat on the floor and your knee approximately over your toes and no further.

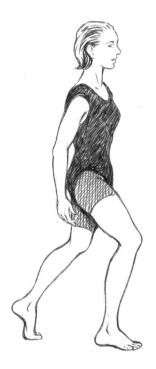

Hold for a count of 1 or 2 and then return to the starting position. As you return, consciously work your right buttock muscle again as you 'push back' into standing.

To progress this exercise further, slowly increase the length of the stride you take, being careful not to over extend your back or lunge too far forward so as to lose your balance.

SCHEDULE:

Repetitions: 5 – 10 times for each leg
Sets: 3
Times per Day: 2 – 3

6) Step Ups

Standing with your left foot on the bottom stair as shown, gently tighten your left buttock muscle and then push through your left leg as you step up to stand with both feet on the same stair.

Once you are standing fully on the stair, gently relax and re-tighten your left buttock muscle as you slowly return to the standing position, leading this time with your right leg.

If you find exercises 4), 5) or 6) too easy, feel free to carry some weights in your hands, e.g. dumbbells, as you perform them. This in effect increases your body weight and therefore the muscles have to work a little harder.

HAMSTRING EXERCISES

1) Bridging

Beginning in the crook lying position, gently tighten your stomach muscles and raise your bottom so it is clear of the surface you are lying on as shown.

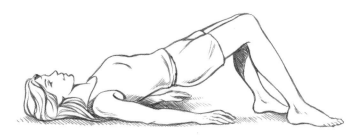

Hold this position for a count of 5-10 seconds and relax. As you find this easy, gradually lift your bottom further from the surface you are lying on, always ensuring your pelvis stays in the neutral position and you do not over-extend your lower back while doing so, especially if you are suffering with EDP. It is also important your body is steady and not wobbling around.

2) Single Leg Bridging

This is similar to the previous bridging exercise, only this time after having tightened your stomach muscles and lifted your bottom from the floor, gently lift one leg from the floor as shown. Hold for 5-10 seconds and return to the crook lying position. Follow this by repeating with your other leg.

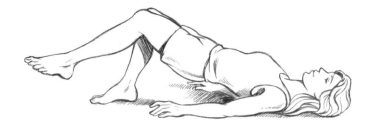

As with the first bridging exercise, if you find this easy, gradually lift your bottom further from the surface you are lying on before raising one foot from the floor, always ensuring your pelvis stays in the neutral position and that your body is steady and not wobbling around.

3) Bridging on a chair

This exercise is similar to the first bridging exercise given on the opposite page, only instead of your feet resting on the floor, have them resting on a small stool/chair. As always, ensure you maintain a neutral spine.

With your feet resting upon the stool/chair, gently tighten your stomach muscles and raise your bottom so it is clear of the surface you are lying on (as shown).

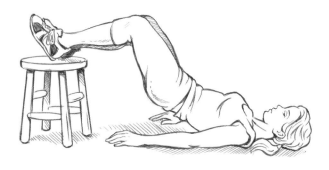

Hold this position for a count of 5-10 seconds and relax. As you find this easy, gradually lift your bottom further from the surface you are lying on, always ensuring your pelvis stays in the neutral position and you do not over-extend your lower back while doing so, especially if you are suffering with EDP. It is also important your body is steady and not wobbling around.

SCHEDULE:

Repetitions: 5 – 10 times
Sets: 3
Times per Day: 2 – 3

N.B. If you feel your Hamstrings begin to 'overwork' with any of the previous bridging exercises, either consciously tighten your Gluteal and Abdominal muscles a little more or lower yourself down and rest. This can happen as a result of the Hamstrings compensating for weak Gluteal muscles, and, if you are not careful, your Hamstring muscles may 'cramp up'.

The important factor to remember when performing the previous three bridging exercises is that once again the lower back and pelvis should maintain a neutral position at all times. In particular with 'single leg bridging' where you are only using one leg to hold your pelvis from the floor, there can be a tendency for one side to deviate or drop down to the side. If this happens, just prior to this is your stopping point. It is important to only take the exercise as far as you can without any asymmetry.

Also, never lift your bottom any higher than it being in line with your chest and thighs.

4) Lunges

While standing, gently tighten your stomach muscles and keep your back straight. Step forward with your left leg as if to start walking. As your foot is about to touch the floor, tighten your left buttock muscle until your foot is flat on the floor and your knee approximately over your toes and no further.

Hold for a count of 1 or 2 and then return to the starting position. As you return, consciously work your left buttock muscle again as you 'push back' into standing.

To progress this exercise further, slowly increase the length of the stride you take, being careful not to over-extend your back or lunge too far forward so as to lose your balance.

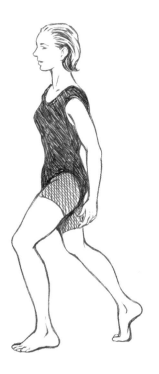

SCHEDULE:

Repetitions: 5 – 10 times for each leg
Sets: 3
Times per Day: 2 – 3

5) Step Ups

Standing with your left foot on the bottom stair as shown, gently tighten your left buttock muscle and then push through your left leg as you step up to stand with both feet on the same stair.

Once you are standing fully on the stair, gently relax and re-tighten your left buttock muscle as you slowly return to the standing position, leading this time with your right leg.

SCHEDULE:

Repetitions: 5 – 10 times for each leg
Sets: 3
Times per Day: 2 – 3

If you find exercise 4) or 5) too easy, feel free to carry some weights in your hands, e.g. dumbbells, as you perform them. This in effect increases your bodyweight and therefore the muscles have to work a little harder.

QUADRICEPS EXERCISES

1) Small Knee Bends

Standing against a wall as shown, gently tighten your stomach and buttock muscles and then slide down the wall. While performing this exercise ensure your hips, knees and second toe are approximately in line with each other and that your hip and knees only bend to a *maximum* of 60 degrees.

When you have lowered yourself to an appropriate level, only hold for a count of 1 or 2 and then slowly raise yourself up again. All the time ensure you are consciously tightening your stomach and Gluteal muscles.

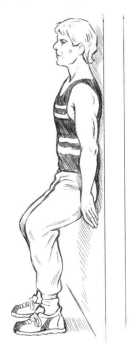

SCHEDULE:

Repetitions: 5 – 10 times
Sets: 3
Times per Day: 1 – 2

267

2) Lunges

While standing, gently tighten your stomach muscles and keep your back straight. Step forward with your left leg as if to start walking. As your foot is about to touch the floor, tighten your left buttock muscle until your foot is flat on the floor and your knee approximately over your toes and no further.

Hold for a count of 1 or 2 and then return to the starting position. As you return, consciously work your left buttock muscle again as you 'push back' into standing.

To progress this exercise further, slowly increase the length of the stride you take, being careful not to over-extend your back or lunge too far forward so as to lose your balance.

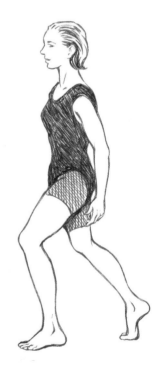

SCHEDULE:

Repetitions: 5 – 10 times for each leg
Sets: 3
Times per Day: 2 – 3

3) Step Ups

Standing with your right foot on the bottom stair as shown, gently tighten your right buttock muscle and then push through your right leg as you step up to stand with both feet on the same stair.

Once you are standing fully on the stair, gently relax and re-tighten your right buttock muscle as you slowly return to the standing position, this time leading with your left leg first.

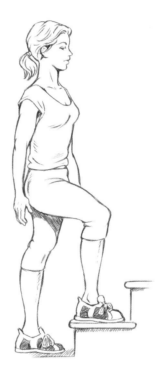

SCHEDULE:

Repetitions: 5 – 10 times for each leg
Sets: 3
Times per Day: 2 – 3

If you find any of the previous exercises 1), 2) or 3) too easy, feel free to carry some weights in your hands, e.g. dumbbells, as you perform them. This in effect increases your bodyweight and therefore the muscles have to work a little harder.

Okay, so you have more or less finished the book now. Just before you do, however, I decided to add one chapter which I thought would be integral to helping those suffering with low back pain and sciatica. That chapter is **Old Wives' Tales.**

I know how frustrating it can be, when everyone you know has an opinion on how to cure yourself of the pain you are suffering. I do not doubt they are telling you the truth, when they say this, that or the other helped them resolve their pain. However, as I am sure you are now more than aware, we are all unique individuals and what helps one person will not necessarily help another. Therefore I thought I would write a chapter on the many old wives' tales I have heard over the years and give you my opinion as to whether there is any validity in them.

Old Wives' Tales

Having spoken to many patients suffering with low back pain and sciatica, I am often told that one of the most frustrating things for them, with the obvious exception of the pain, is that everyone has an opinion on what they should and should not do.

I'm sure you are familiar with what I am going to say… a work colleague may recommend physiotherapy/osteopathy/chiropractic (delete as applicable) or maybe a friend will tell you how you must try acupuncture, as it worked wonders for him or her. There will also be those that swear by Cod Liver Oil, Glucosamine, other oils, tiger balm, back stretchers, orthopaedic beds, memory foam mattresses, massaging machines… the list is probably endless.

What I hope to do by writing this chapter is help you out with regard to my experience and knowledge as to which old wives' tales are worth pursuing and which ones are not. I will have to put my little 'disclaimer' in here though. I'm sure you must know this by now…ultimately, *listen to your body!* If you try something and it aggravates your pain, it is not working for you so therefore ease off. On the other hand, if it eases your pain, feel free to continue.

Let's say, for example, I have been seeing someone for three treatments and he is getting no better. When he arrives for his fourth appointment he informs me he is 75 per cent better and has been so ever since he began taking his mother's secret remedy of this, that and the other.

Am I then going to say stop taking it, as it has nothing to do with his pain improving? No way. Whether or not I feel it has improved his pain, if he is convinced it has helped, and therefore wants to continue taking it, I'm going to say, "By all means, carry on." (As long as I feel it is not being detrimental to his general health!)

It is important that I add, however, I would still encourage him to work on any particular exercises which would resolve his last 25 per cent and also, probably more importantly, reduce the chances of him suffering with pain again in the future.

Is there a chance this patient's mother's remedy was helping him due to the placebo effect? There is a fair probability it is. Is that a problem? I do not think so. Some health professionals mock the placebo effect and say that certain treatments are only that. Well, let me ask you, if you went to see a practitioner and were treated with what medical science would say has only a placebo effect, and yet it cured you of your pain, would you care? I think I know the answer to that one.

Without any shadow of doubt the placebo effect works. You only have to look at almost any medical research that takes place. Half of the group are typically given the infamous 'sugar tablet' placebo as a control group and yet some of them will undoubtedly get better.

As health professionals, if we could find out how the placebo effect works… WOW! Whoever discovered it would be up for a Nobel Prize in Medicine, I'm sure. It would be the biggest breakthrough in medicine ever! Unfortunately, no one has and I do not suppose they ever will.

My drawn-out point here is that if it works don't knock it, take advantage of it. However, I would also suggest you bear in mind the fundamental principles of this book and remove as many inappropriate stresses from your back as possible as well because ultimately, whether the placebo effect worked or not, *it is imperative we get to what we feel is the cause of the pain in the first place*.

I will now go on to outline a few of what I consider to be old wives' tales and give you my opinion on them. Just remember though, this is only *my opinion* and if through your experience you disagree, that's fine.

Once you have suffered with low back pain or sciatica, you will always suffer with it

I hope you know the answer to this one. If you do not, I will say here without doubt I strongly believe this **NOT** to be true. To understand why, please read the chapter, **Learning Zone: *Why Muscles are the Key Factor in Eliminating Your Pain.***

Wearing a back support will weaken the muscles in your back

This is not too difficult to answer, yet I need to be careful how I say it. First, I am not a great lover of these as I feel in the majority of cases they are not necessary. If we correct our postures and activities as appropriate, along with a prescribed exercise programme, our own muscles and ligaments are more than capable of supporting our lower back. Therefore, a back support is not necessary.

However, there may be times when your pain is so severe or you are unable to avoid certain aggravating activities, for example due to work, that your back needs some kind of extra support. In such circumstances I would say it is okay to use one.

However, the statement was that using a back support would make your back weak. Is that true? I have to say I do not believe this to be true, as long as you use the support sensibly. If you were to use it twenty-four hours a day, day-in, day-out, then there is every chance this may encourage the stabilising muscles about your back to become lazy and switch off a little.

However, if you were to wear it only during the activities with which you felt your back needed some extra support, yet outside of these activities not only did you remove the support but also performed some exercises to increase the stability of your back, then go ahead, that's fine. In actual fact I would go as far as to say it is the sensible thing to do.

I say this because you would be preventing your back from being aggravated by providing it with the extra support (and you should know I am a great advocate of anything that reduces aggravating factors). Yet you would also be actively exercising the stabilising muscles about your back when not using the support, thereby encouraging the back to become stronger and reducing the need for extra support in the long term.

Placing a pillow in the small of your back will help when you are sitting

To say whether I agree with this statement in one word, I would have to say 'Yes', there would have to be a little caveat though. As a rule of thumb this will be a good thing to do as it would help support the natural curve of the lower back, which we refer to as lordosis, see the chapter, **Learning Zone:** *Your Lower Back and Sciatic Nerve*. However, there could be a couple of drawbacks when doing this:

i) **If the pillow is too big and therefore doesn't fit nicely into the curve of your back.**

This could actually push you forward on the chair as opposed to supporting your back. This in turn could encourage you effectively to be leaning forward and therefore placing a flexion stress upon your back.

ii) **If the pillow fits the curve in your back nicely, but is too 'fat or round'.**

This could accentuate the lordotic curve in your back. This in particular could be a problem for someone suffering with EDP.

You can buy lumbar supports from a number of shops or online. Personally, I get on well with these. However, I do know of people who do not because they find them too big and feel they are being pushed forward. I can also relate to this. I just correct my sitting accordingly and maybe do not push my bottom quite 100 per cent back into the chair.

For those who do not like them, I often recommend they use a small, rolled-up towel as this can be just as effective. If you were to use something like this, simply roll it up to the size which you find most comfortable, place an elastic band or something similar around each end and leave it on any chair which you tend to use, including your car seat. Every time you then go to sit down, it is there waiting for you.

For further information on sitting and what I feel are the best principles to bear in mind when doing so, read the chapter, **Practical Advice:** *The Influence of Regular Day-to-day Activities on Your Pain.*

It's because you are overweight that you are in pain

Not necessarily, although it does increase the chances of you developing low back pain or sciatica, as well as decrease the chances of you resolving your pain. A fair amount of this is due to your particular make-up. As I have mentioned several times throughout this book, we are all born differently and our bodies cope with increased stresses in different ways. I know of a few people who are significantly overweight and yet they have never suffered with any kind of low back pain or sciatica, just as I have treated plenty of people who are not overweight yet they are suffering with low back pain or sciatica.

The simple truth of it, as far as I am concerned, is that if you are overweight you will be placing increased stresses across your back. If you are placing increased stresses across your back this will increase the *likelihood* of you developing pain, or, if you already have pain, decrease the chances of you curing yourself of that pain. It goes without saying that the more overweight you are, the greater the stress across your back and therefore the greater the consequences of that.

If you know you are overweight and are suffering with low back pain or sciatica, losing weight will help contribute to resolving your pain.

Taking anti-inflammatories will only mask your pain

Once again, you are probably aware by now that I am not an advocate of taking medication for the sake of it. However, I do believe anti-inflammatories can play an important temporary role in the treatment of low back pain or sciatica.

My approach to low back pain and sciatica is all about the re-education of incorrect postures along with appropriate stretching and strengthening exercises. If, due to acutely inflamed pain, you are prevented from performing these exercises, I would say the use of anti-inflammatories should be encouraged (providing there are no contra-indications).

This would not be masking the pain, but rather settling down the sensitivity of the pain to enable you to exercise more. By exercising more, your back would become stronger and more supple, which in turn would help decrease the inflammation present and therefore ease your pain.

If I can refer you back to **Step Two:** *How to STOP Acutely Inflamed Pain* you will see in more detail why I believe anti-inflammatories can be an integral part of your treatment.

If you are not sleeping well you need to replace your bed

I'm afraid I have to disagree wholeheartedly with this statement. More often than not, if you are not sleeping well, it is due to the position you are sleeping in or what you were up to before you went to bed that is the problem, not the bed itself. If I can refer you back to the chapter, **Practical Advice:** *Do Not Replace Your Bed* and encourage you to read this before you even think about replacing your bed.

Taking supplements such as Cod Liver Oil and Glucosamine will help resolve your pain

I'm afraid I am going to well and truly sit on the fence with this one. Research has taken place regarding the use of supplements such as these, but the results seem to be inconclusive when looked at as a whole. In addition to this, the feedback I have had from patients regarding numerous different supplements is also inconclusive. I would say if you are going to try these, you need really to try them for about three months before you can decide whether they are working. All I can add to that, is if after this time you feel they are working, then feel free to continue taking them. If however you feel no different, you may as well stop…sorry, not much help there I'm afraid!

Swimming is good exercise for a bad back

This depends on why you are suffering with your pain and the type of swimming stroke you tend to use. Firstly, I would say if you are suffering with acutely inflamed pain, the chances are that swimming with any stroke is likely to aggravate it. I would therefore suggest you read **Step Two:**

How to STOP Acutely Inflamed Pain. If, however, your pain has settled somewhat and you are able to perform some significant exercise, feel free to try swimming but still be careful. A lot will depend upon the diagnosis you have given yourself and also which stroke you intend to use.

FRONT CRAWL/FREESTYLE

As this is performed in the 'prone' position, you should not be surprised when I say it may aggravate someone with EDP, although not quite as much as when simply lying on the floor/bed, as the buoyancy gained from the water will help decrease the effect of gravity on the spine.

BREAST STROKE

This will also tend to aggravate the person suffering with EDP, as not only are you in the prone position similar to front crawl/freestyle, but you will also be actively extending your spine with each stroke. As a result of this active extension, this stroke will tend to aggravate EDP more than front crawl/freestyle.

BUTTERFLY

Like the breast stroke, this is performed in the prone position and therefore has an element of extension. It also involves active extension as your head comes out of the water. Consequently, this may well aggravate EDP.

BACK STROKE

This stroke will probably be the only one that someone with EDP may like, as it will not naturally encourage the lower back into extension. However, if you have EDP as a result of tight hip flexors or Latissimus Dorsi muscle, your back could be aggravated as a result of:

i)   Tight hip flexors (Quadriceps and Iliopsoas) forcing your low back into extension due to you being in the supine position.

ii)   Tight Latissimus Dorsi muscle forcing your back into extension as you take your arms above your head.

For further explanations on how these muscles will have such an effect, please read the chapter, **Learning Zone:** *Why Muscles are the Key Factor in Eliminating Your Pain.*

Remember, those activities which tend to aggravate one diagnosis, as a rule of thumb, will tend to ease the opposite diagnosis. Therefore, with the above swimming strokes, if I have stated it is likely to aggravate EDP, there is a reasonable chance it will ease FDP and vice versa. Be careful, however, as you will be giving your back a significant amount of exercise… and you can get too much of a good thing!

A little caution should always be taken when swimming for the first time. As a rule of thumb it is a good exercise, as it works practically all of the body and is also a non-weight-bearing exercise. However, do not be led into a false sense of security. By this, I mean it is not uncommon for people to tell me they tried some swimming and although it felt great while they were in the pool, they really suffered afterwards.

I feel the reason for this is that the buoyancy of the water helps take pressure from the back and, particularly if the water is warm, helps relax muscles and therefore loosens them up. It is therefore no surprise that your pain may feel better at first. However, you are still giving your back quite a bit of exercise, yet under these comforting conditions you may not be given a warning your pain is being aggravated until you are out of the pool and have 'cooled down'.

This is why I say if you are to try swimming, judge for yourself *before you go in* how much you feel your pain will be able to tolerate and then stick to it. If, while you are swimming, your pain becomes a little aggravated before you have reached you original aim, it is time to stop. On the other hand, if you have reached your target and your pain feels fine *it is still time to get out.* This is so you do not fall into the trap of overdoing it without noticing.

If, after you have carried on with your day, you feel no adverse reaction, then great. The next time you go swimming do the same again or maybe even try a little more. If, on the other hand, you notice within an hour or so that the swimming did aggravate your pain, you know you need to at least ease off the next time you go back, or depending upon how sore your pain was, maybe give swimming a miss for a little while until your body has healed itself further.

You need to rest/keep active if you want your pain to get better

I have seen very contrasting attitudes with regard to whether resting or keeping active is a good thing for your low back pain/sciatica. The majority of people who get this wrong tend to over-rest, either through fear of doing further damage or because they have been given incorrect information by someone else.

On the other hand, I have also treated patients who have been advised that it is important to keep active and have therefore continued to soldier on with their day-to-day activities even though it has been aggravating their pain no end.

In general, the advice to keep active is sound; however, sometimes it is easier said than done. Under such circumstances, complete rest can be indicated for a day or two. I will refer you to **Step Two: *How to STOP Acutely Inflamed Pain*** as this will explain the best way to achieve complete rest. As a rule of thumb though, this should be for no longer than 36-48 hours, and then you must try to become active no matter how little that activity may be.

Use warmth/cold for your back

Once again, I have experienced contrasting reports as to what patients prefer; warmth or cold. In theory, I would say warmth is best for most backs. This is due to the warmth helping to increase blood flow and relax the area, especially if there are tight muscles present. Cold, on the other hand, gives the opposite effect by decreasing the blood flow and causing the area to tighten up.

The only time I would suggest cold over warmth is if the individual concerned has an acutely inflamed back, typically the first 36-48 hours after injury. If you were to use warmth during this stage, it could inflame things further. After this, however, I would lean towards warmth or nothing at all as being appropriate.

However, I am sure you can guess what I am going to say now…listen to your body. I have treated some patients, although not many, with chronic long-term back problems who say that warmth aggravates their pain and cold eases it. Am I going to ask them to use warmth as the theory says it should be best? Of course I am not, as their pain obviously disagrees! Your body knows what it likes best, therefore be guided by it.

If you feel uncomfortable, just fidget about

I'm afraid not. The typical example here is sitting. Many people feel they need to fidget if they have been sitting for too long. How long is too long? When your pain increases. I do not want you to fidget at all.

DOES THAT MEAN YOU JUST HAVE TO SIT THERE?

Absolutely not. If you feel the need to fidget, that is your body telling you it is fed up with being in that position, therefore change it. If you have been sitting, that means stand up and have a little walk around, even if it's only for half a minute or so. I'm sure you are aware that if you do fidget it only gives you momentary relief and then you will begin fidgeting again. What you need to do is change your posture/position.

Another classic 'fidgeting' posture is standing. Once again, try not to fidget around by transferring your weight from leg to leg; instead, go for a little walk if practical or maybe even sit down…not for too long though. If I can refer you back to the chapter, **Practical Advice: *The Influence of Regular Day-to-day Activities on Your Pain*** for a more in-depth discussion regarding sitting and standing and its effects on your pain.

Once you have had low back pain/sciatica, you will never again be able to return to vigorous exercise or the gym

I'm hoping you know my answer to this statement. Of course you will, but that doesn't mean a level of caution should not be taken when returning again or starting for the first time. Probably the most important advice I can give you with regard to this, apart from listening to your body, is to be very aware of the neutral posture of your spine.

Remember, if you put increased stresses across your back and your back does not have the stability to support it, it will deviate from that neutral posture and increase the chances of you developing pain again. Examples of this include trying to lift too heavy a weight or if you are running and begin to fatigue.

If there is one thing I would really encourage you to do when your pain eases, it would be to take up some form of exercise; you will only benefit from it. However, be sensible and ease yourself into the given exercise and ultimately...*listen to your body!*

No Pain – No Gain

This is definitely a big myth I would like to bust. As far as I am concerned, if you are doing something and it is resulting in increased pain, you are interfering with the healing process. Therefore you will definitely be getting no 'gain' from it at all.

We need to set up the optimal conditions for your body to heal itself, which means putting optimal stresses across it in order for it to heal well and strong, but not excess stresses that will prevent or disrupt the healing process.

Leave the 'No Pain – No Gain' approach to the muscle-bound folk in the gym, not for when the body is trying to heal itself! For a more in-depth discussion on why I take this approach, read the chapter, **Learning Zone:** *Your Own Body is the Greatest Healer* and **Step Three:** *How to Optimise Your Body's Healing Potential.*

If it hurts, it means you are causing long-term damage

This is simply not true. If you are going about your normal day-to-day activities or performing certain exercises given throughout this book, it is virtually impossible to cause any significant long-term damage to your back. Having said that, this does not mean you may not make your pain a little worse every now and again.

If you are feeling pain for whatever reason, this is simply the body's way of telling you to ease off a little, as you are placing excess stress across the injured structures and are therefore interfering with your body's healing process. If you heed this warning, your pain will soon settle down. Once the pain has settled, ask yourself what you may have been doing to aggravate your pain.

If you feel it was a day-to-day activity that aggravated your pain, I would ask you temporarily to avoid or modify that activity if possible. If, on the other hand, it was an exercise given from this book, I would ask you to ease off initially on that particular exercise before thinking about disregarding it completely.

If, however, you continue to ease off and it still aggravates your pain, then feel free to disregard it for the time being and drop back to a level which you know you are comfortable with.

For further information regarding this topic, please read the following chapters – **Learning Zone:** *Your Own Body is the Greatest Healer,* **Step Three:** *How to Optimise Your Body's Healing Potential* and **Learning Zone:** *The Principles of Exercise.*

I always emphasise the following point to people when this subject arises:

Learn to respect pain, but never be fearful of it

Yes, your body will give you pain for a reason, but it is simply a warning sign that something is not right. Therefore respect the fact you are being given such a message and act accordingly, the pain will then soon disappear. However, do not be fearful of pain and frightened to do anything at all.

If you need to rest your back, just sit down

Please do not do this. In actual fact, for a lot of low back pain and sciatica, sitting down can be one of the most stressful things you can do. I have treated many patients who, as a result of their pain, have felt they are resting it by sitting down all day or maybe lying in bed watching TV. Nothing could be further from the truth.

Do not get me wrong, there are a few occasions when an acute attack of pain may dictate a day or two's rest, but even then there is an emphasis on keeping as active as possible – see **Step Two:** *How to STOP Acutely Inflamed Pain*. In addition to this, resting your back means placing the appropriate amount of stress across your back, not as little stress as possible.

It is important you place increased stresses across your back as it heals so it will heal stronger. It is equally important though that these stresses are not excessive as they will interfere with the body's healing process. By placing the appropriate stresses across your back, it will be resting but also healing with strength. Please read **Step Five:** *Getting Moving Again* and also the chapter, **Practical Advice:** *The Influence of Regular Day-to-day Activities on Your Pain* for further information.

It's because you are unfit that your muscles are tight

Another false statement. Fitness has nothing to do with your muscles being tight. If anything, the opposite can sometimes be true. I have had many people visit me in the physiotherapy department who are extremely fit and go running and go to the gym regularly, yet they never stretch out. Their muscles and back can be as stiff as a board.

Any time at all after exercise, it is important to stretch out the muscles you have been using otherwise they will be liable to tighten up. This is why you will always see conditioned athletes stretching.

Anti-inflammatory gels will help your pain

I'm afraid I am not a great lover of these, simply because experience tells me they offer only temporary relief at best. You will be aware I am an advocate of taking anti-inflammatory tablets, where the anti-inflammatory can get into your system and address the inflammation taking place. However, I am not so convinced with regard to these topical agents. If you have used them and are grateful for any temporary relief you may receive, then great, feel free to continue. However, I would be surprised if you gain any more benefit than that.

Your spine or pelvis is 'out' / 'rotated' / 'twisted', etc. and needs to be 'put back in'

Sorry, but I do not believe in this school of thought. I often hear patients say they have been told this is the problem with their back, and also that it will need subsequent regular treatments for it to be 'corrected' or 'put back in'. As I have said a number of times in this book, we are all unique individuals, and there are probably more of us that do not adhere to the pure anatomical model which we see printed in books than there are those that do.

My point here is that sure, there maybe one or two of us with a slightly rotated spine or pelvis. Is this the cause of the pain, however? I'm more than likely to think it is not specifically this that is causing you pain, but rather the stresses being placed across those structures which are the problem.

By this, I mean it could be these increased stresses that are creating the slight 'mal-alignment' or that these stresses are causing your pain threshold levels to be breached. Either way, it is these stresses which we need to address.

Besides, I would say it is very difficult to simply 'manipulate' a joint back into place – just because you may hear or feel a 'crack' when being treated definitely does not mean that the joint has moved 'back in'. Also, even if it could be clicked back in that easy, who is to say it isn't going to move out again once we get back to our day-to-day activities? This further reinforces the need to address any particular tight or weak structures which have an influence on that particular joint and therefore may be causing the mal-alignment.

Massage will help ease your pain

Of all the hands-on treatment I still perform, I personally find this to be the most beneficial. Although it may be the joints of the back or the discs which are causing you pain, it is more often than not the soft tissues, and in particular the muscles, that are exerting the stresses across these structures and therefore resulting in your pain. Massage has been found to decrease pain and stress as well as increase blood flow and encourage tight muscles to relax. This will all help them to function correctly.

I will have to add, though, the answer to your pain is unlikely to be simply massage. If, for example, you have muscles that are tight and they are the cause of your pain, then I have no doubt massage will help. However, we still need to address the reasons as to why these muscles were tight in the first place. If you do not address this, there is every chance your pain will feel better for a while afterwards, but it will soon reappear as the muscles tighten up again.

Therefore, by all means book yourself in for a massage somewhere, but still use the principles given throughout this book in order to address the cause of your tight muscles, as well as stretch the tight structures out regularly.

One word of caution; I would probably advise against massage if your pain is in the extremely acute inflammatory stage (see **Step Two:** *How to STOP Acutely Inflamed Pain*) as it would probably aggravate your pain.

One leg being longer than the other or flat feet is probably the cause of your pain

It's time for me to sit on the fence again. The precise reply to this statement is that either can lead to low back pain or sciatica. The question you need to ask yourself is "Is it causing *my* pain?"

The reason I say this is because I have treated some patients where this has been a cause of their pain, but others where even though they may have had a leg-length discrepancy/flat feet, it was not the cause of their pain.

As I have alluded to before, the body is a wonderful compensator and will put up with many stresses without causing any pain at all. Therefore it is important not to be complacent and just 'assume' that because there is a leg-length discrepancy or flat feet present it is automatically the cause of the pain.

To begin with, the best way to find out whether it may be influencing your pain is to ask yourself some further questions. The first one would be with regard to your aggravating and easing factors...

DOES SITTING AGGRAVATE YOUR PAIN?

If sitting is one of the worst things you can do for your low back pain or sciatica and walking around eases your pain, it is very unlikely your leg length or flat feet have anything to do with your pain. If you think about it, one leg could be six inches longer than the other but it matters nothing to your back if you are sitting down.

The only time either of these two are going to have an influence on your pain is when you are on your feet, be it standing or walking. If these activities do not aggravate your pain, it is unlikely they are the cause of your pain.

If the opposite is true and walking and/or standing does aggravate your pain, then these factors *may* be having a causative effect. The operative word here is 'may' as it may also be a red herring.

If it is flat feet you have and you feel they may be the cause of your pain, the next question you need to ask yourself is...

DOES MY PAIN FEEL BETTER OR WORSE IN CERTAIN FOOTWEAR COMPARED TO OTHERS?

If there is certain footwear you prefer with regard to your pain, have a look inside and see if they have a significant arch support compared to the ones you are not so keen on wearing. If so, there is a likelihood (and it is still only a likelihood) that you may need some support for the arches of your feet.

Arch supports are incredibly expensive if you were to visit a podiatrist and have them custom made, especially if you consider they may make no difference at all to your pain. I would suggest that at first you try buying some 'off the shelf' orthotics for your shoes. These should say on the packaging that they are for flat feet, dropped arches or over-pronation. They may also be referred to as 'medial arch supports'.

In particular, there are orthotics out there that offer a 30-day money back guarantee when you purchase them. Try these for a few weeks to see if they help. If they help then great; if not, the chances are your arches are not a cause for concern so go back to the shop and get your money back! If they help a little, then the choice is yours as to whether you have some custom-made ones; this may be the answer to your problems, but then again it may not...

If you feel you have a leg-length discrepancy, try finding a small amount of felt, or purchasing an off-the-shelf heel raise, and place it in the heel of the shoe of your shorter leg. Walk around for a few days and see if it makes any difference to your pain. If it helps, once again there is a fair chance this may be contributing to your pain. This could be enough to sort your problem out, in which case make sure you place a heel raise in all of your shoes for the short leg.

> *Remember, whether you are placing a heel raise or arch support in your shoe, it should not aggravate your pain. If it does, remove it completely or modify it a little.*
> *Having said that, it is not unusual for people to say their feet or calves ache a little after placing orthotics in their shoes. This is nothing to worry about and is likely to be a result of the muscles working a little differently in response to the changes taking place. If it is only a little bit achy, you may wish to bear with it. However, if it is too uncomfortable, feel free to remove the orthotic every few hours, in order to give your leg some rest but also familiarise it with the change taking place.*

You should expect and accept pain if you are 'old'

Absolutely not! The body will continue to heal itself as long as you are alive. Therefore, if you are alive enough to feel pain, you are alive enough for your body to heal itself of that pain!

Now I am not going to try and kid you and say your body will heal itself the same as it did when you were twenty-one; it isn't, and I'm sure you know that anyway. As we get older the body isn't as efficient at healing itself compared to when we were younger, but nevertheless it will still try.

In addition to this, we are going to have more wear and tear present as we get older, which itself increases the ***chances*** of feeling pain (see 'Arthritis' in **Appendix I: *Glossary of Diagnostic Terms***).

Also, the likelihood is we are not as mobile as we were when we were younger, which once again can contribute to the chances of feeling pain. However, all of the above factors simply increase the ***chances*** of developing pain; they do not mean you will get pain or if you do that you should just accept it…definitely not!

As I mentioned earlier, as long as you are alive your body will try to heal itself. Therefore, bear in mind the principles of this book and provide yourself with an appropriate exercise programme…you may surprise yourself as you find your pain eases away.

Taking a hot bath will ease your pain

This is a question I am often asked and I am sure you know what the answer is going to be again… . How does your pain respond to taking a hot bath? I have mentioned numerous times before, everyone really is different and therefore it is imperative you listen to how *your* body, and in particular *your* pain, responds to any of your day-to-day activities.

I will now give a few examples as to why taking a hot bath may be particularly beneficial, or not so, as the case may be.

One of the main reasons why a hot bath may help your pain is primarily due to the warmth. By spending some time 'soaking' in a bath, the warmth is going to penetrate the deeper muscles, which in turn will increase blood flow to the area and help the muscles relax. Therefore, particularly if you are suffering with EDP, which is a result of tight soft tissues, there is a very good chance you will find taking a nice hot bath beneficial.

However, taking a hot bath can also have its downside. One of the likely aggravating factors is your position. From your waist down you will be pretty straight, but from the waist up you will be lying back, in a kind of 'reclined' sitting position. This will be putting a flexion stress across your back not dissimilar to sitting slumped. You will therefore understand how spending any length of time in a hot bath could potentially aggravate someone's pain who is suffering with FDP.

However, if I refer you back to the analogy of bending your finger back in **Step Four:** *How to Diagnose Your Pain*, you will see how it could also aggravate someone's pain who is suffering with EDP.

In this situation, the warmth of the bath can lead you into a false sense of security, in that it feels relaxing and may ease your pain while in the bath; however, it may begin to overstretch your muscles without you realising it. This would normally take the pattern of your pain still feeling eased immediately after getting out of the bath, but a little while afterwards the pain beginning to increase and your back stiffening or tightening up.

I will use a clinical example which highlights this point well and also reinforces the point that if your pain feels particularly better or worse, you always need to ask yourself what you may have been doing to have created this situation.

I was treating a patient who returned to the physiotherapy department stating that although she felt her pain was generally getting better, she had recently found it difficult to get to sleep and was waking during the night as a result of increased pain.

My first thought was to ask her what she had been doing the previous evening that may have been aggravating her pain. Had she been spending too long sitting without standing up, performing housework, etc? To all of these questions she was adamant she had done nothing different.

On further questioning however, she did mention in passing that she had started to take a bath before she went to bed. I asked her how her pain was as a result of this, to which she replied, "Lovely." On further questioning, however, it became apparent that although her pain did feel 'lovely' while she was in the bath, now she thought about it, it did feel worse a little while after she had got out of the bath and got herself ready for bed.

Bearing in mind the only thing that had changed with regard to her sleep being okay and her sleep not being okay was her taking a bath, I felt we were onto something as to why her sleep was now a problem.

I discussed this with her, to which she replied something along the lines of, "Oh, I thought taking a hot bath would be good for my pain, and it felt so nice while I was in there." My obvious reply to this was to remind her of the principle that if your pain feels particularly better or worse you need to ask yourself:

"What am I doing now and what have I been doing for the last hour or so?"

If she had done this straight away, she would have identified the bath as a possible aggravating factor. She could therefore have stopped taking the hot bath before bed for a day or two to see if this made any difference. This is exactly what I asked her to do, and within a few days her sleeping was fine again.

I know this last section was about whether a hot bath is good for your pain, and in answer to that question I would say as a rule of thumb it can be beneficial for someone with EDP (although try not to spend too long in there), but to be careful if you are suffering with FDP. However, I would also like to use this example to reinforce the principles given throughout this book, and that is that no health professional or book can give you a definitive answer to any question as to what is good or not so good for your pain.

Ultimately, you need to *listen to your body*. I have seen far too many people who have presented themselves with similar signs and symptoms and have been given a similar diagnosis, yet what would ease one of their pains would aggravate another's.

I hope this chapter has guided you through the likelihood of what is good or not so good for your pain with regard to some classic old wives' tales. Ultimately, always remember…

listen to your body, as your body will soon tell you whether what you are doing is good or not so good for it!

Conclusion

Congratulations and thank you for completing this book. If you are suffering with low back pain or sciatica at the moment, I understand how you are feeling. I have treated many, many patients who are struggling to go to work or about their day-to-day activities because of this type of pain.

As I have alluded to many times throughout this book, the body really is fantastic at repairing and healing itself, and if you adopt the principles and appropriate exercises given, your body will begin to cure itself of your pain.

I appreciate and fully understand there will be some small sacrifices to be made along the way; maybe you won't be able to sit in your favourite soft chair for a while or you may have to give yourself a small break from gardening. However, any activities that this book suggests you modify or avoid will only be those which are increasing your pain anyway, and therefore consequently preventing it from getting better.

These small sacrifices will only be temporary because if your body is given the correct conditions in which to heal itself, then heal itself it will. Following this, it should not be long before you are carrying out those activities once again, only this time with no pain whatsoever.

On the flip side of these small sacrifices, I have treated many patients who have started exercising as a result of the advice I have given them, and they have found themselves enjoying it so much they have continued to do so even after their pain has completely resolved itself.

This has varied from people joining a gym and becoming quite active, to simply going for regular walks. Either way, exercise is a fantastic way of keeping healthy and fighting off many aches and pains. If this book results in you being one of those individuals, then fantastic, you will without doubt benefit from the rewards of this.

As you go about incorporating the principles of this book into your lifestyle, you may be quite lucky and make just a few relatively straightforward changes as to how you are carrying out your day-to-day activities and it will be enough for your pain to resolve itself completely. On the other hand, you may have to work a little harder and perform a few more exercises, and also be very analytical about those things that are preventing your body from healing itself of the pain you are suffering.

If you are one of the latter, all I can do is urge you to be patient. It may be a little frustrating at first, but you will get there. Stick with it and you will reap the rewards as your pain begins to disappear.

Thank you once again for reading this book and remember, you possess within yourself the most wonderful and fantastic healing capabilities known to man...

If you look after and listen to your own body, it will look after you.

Take Care and Good Luck.

Paul

Appendix I:

Glossary of Diagnostic Terms

I know how frustrating it can be to be given a diagnosis by a GP or Consultant only to arrive home and not have a clue what they have been talking about. Any diagnosis should be clearly explained. This chapter does just that. I will give a list of all the typical diagnostic terms which are given for low back pain or sciatica and then explain them in lay terms. Where appropriate I have given an informative website address regarding these conditions, so you are able to research any further information should you wish to.

Ankylosing Spondylitis (AS)

Website: <http://www.nass.co.uk>
Ankylosing Spondylitis is a progressive, rheumatic disease which affects mainly the spine, although it can also affect other joints such as the hips and knees. It can also influence other soft tissues such as tendons and ligaments.

Its typical signs and symptoms are a slow gradual onset of pain and stiffness, over months or years as opposed to hours or days.

If you feel you may be suffering with AS, I would first recommend you research the condition further. The National Ankylosing Spondylitis Society (NASS) is an excellent source for further information. If you still feel you may be suffering with this then I suggest you visit your GP.

If you have been diagnosed with AS, it is important you are referred to a rheumatologist for the diagnosis to be confirmed and appropriate medication prescribed. It is then important you are referred to a physiotherapist to be given a suitable exercise programme.

Arthritis

Website: <http://www.arc.org.uk>
Arthritis, when literally broken down, means: joint (arthro), inflammation (itis). This term is synonymous with Osteo-Arthritis.

Arthritis is wear and tear and we will all suffer from this as we get older. When I say older, some people will begin to show degrees of wear and tear in their spine from as young as their late twenties! Therefore, if you receive the results of your x-ray and you are told you have wear and tear/

Arthritis/Osteo-Arthritis/Spondylosis, etc. of the spine, do not be too concerned and think there is nothing which can be done for your pain.

The reason for me highlighting this is that I see many patients who tell me they know why they are suffering with low back pain or sciatica; it is because they have arthritis of the spine. They sometimes go on to tell me they do not know why they have been referred for physiotherapy as 'you cannot do anything for arthritis'.

Usually my first response to this is, "Yes, you are right, there is absolutely nothing I can do about the arthritis you have." I then quickly follow this statement up with, "However, that doesn't mean we can do nothing about the pain you are suffering."

As we get older and suffer wear and tear of any joint, this only means the **chances** of us developing pain from that joint have increased; it is not a foregone conclusion, however.

As the wear and tear occurs, physical changes take place about that joint in response to the increased stresses placed across it. It is how our body adapts to these changes which is the biggest influence on whether or not we will suffer pain, not the changes themselves.

Some people are very fortunate in that their x-rays may show a high degree of wear and tear present, yet they may be suffering very little or no pain at all. On the other hand, another person may not be so fortunate and have an x-ray showing the arthritic changes present are relatively small, yet they will be in quite severe pain. The main difference between these two individuals is not relative to the amount of wear and tear present, but rather how their bodies have responded to that wear and tear.

The most significant thing arthritis does to a joint is that it sensitises the structures involved, consequently increasing the **likelihood** of perceiving pain. Therefore, if we can reduce the stresses across the joints concerned – this may be by either stretching or strengthening the appropriate structures that have an influence over the arthritic joint, or simply by making some postural adjustments (all of which are covered in this book) – there is every chance we can decrease the pain.

I appreciate I have been a bit long-winded with this, but my point is that if you are suffering with low back pain or sciatica as a result of arthritis, do not give up hope. Although it may be a little more difficult, it does not necessarily mean there is nothing which can be done for you. I have treated many patients who have been diagnosed with arthritis of their spine, yet they have gone on to make a 100 per cent recovery, so there is no reason why you too should not be able to.

In addition to this, it is important I add that the arthritis shown by the x-ray may be a red herring and have nothing at all to do with your pain. Bearing in mind the majority of us will show signs of arthritis in our spine as we pass through our late twenties/thirties, if you were to x-ray 100 people in this age group who were suffering with no pain whatsoever, there is a very high likelihood that some of these x-rays will show signs of arthritis in their spine. So why do they not have low back pain or sciatica?

The reason is, as I have explained above, arthritis increases the likelihood of you getting pain, it does not mean you are going to suffer pain. Even though you may be showing signs of arthritis on your x-ray, there may be another, more simple reason, for the pain you are suffering, which has nothing to do with arthritis.

All I am saying is that if you have been told you have arthritis of your spine, do not be too alarmed. It is something everyone will have as they get older and may have nothing at all to do with your pain. Even if it does, it can be treated appropriately in order to resolve the pain.

Arthropathy

If you were to look this up in a dictionary, it would probably tell you it is joint disease (anything with 'arthro' in it always refers to the joint). However, do not be perturbed by the word disease, it usually means there is something wrong with the joint, this may simply be wear and tear (see Arthritis).

Cauda Equina Syndrome (CES)

Website: <http://www.caudaequina.org/definition.html>
<http://www.oldcity.org.uk/cauda_equina>

At approximately the level of the first/second lumbar vertebra, the spinal cord itself finishes and the nerves form a group together referred to as the Cauda Equina. This is Latin for horse's tail, which it is said to resemble. If there is any kind of compression on the nerves in this region, typically by a prolapsed disc, it does not allow these nerves to function correctly. Typical signs and symptoms you would present with if this were the case are as follows:

a) **Decreased Bladder and Bowel Control**
   The group of nerves concerned provide you with conscious control over your bladder and bowel movements. If for any reason you feel you have decreased control over your bladder or bowel, you may be suffering with CES. These symptoms may include difficulty emptying your bladder or bowel or the opposite where you find it difficult to stop yourself from emptying your bladder or bowel.

b) **Saddle Paraesthesia (numbness and/or pins and needles)**
   These same nerves also provide you with sensation between your legs, or what is often referred to as the 'saddle' area. You may feel numbness or pins and needles in this area, i.e. in between the legs, genitalia, inner thigh or buttock area. Some people have described how it feels 'funny' or 'different' when they wipe themselves after having been to the toilet.

c) **Pain in the saddle area**
   This same saddle area, where you can suffer with paraesthesia, may also be a region where you suffer pain.

d) **Sexual Dysfunction**
   This could be in the form of impotence or loss of ejaculation/orgasm.

If you feel you may be suffering with CES, it is important you seek ***immediate medical advice.*** Contact your GP immediately and inform him or her of your signs and symptoms and wait for advice as to the next step you should take. If, for whatever reason, you are unable to speak to your GP, visit your local A&E department.

Severe pain and subsequent medication can also give similar signs and symptoms to CES, for example:

i)   If you are suffering with intense low back pain, it is sometimes difficult to go to the toilet as even the simplest strain will increase your pain.

ii) Some pain-relieving medication can result in quite severe constipation, resulting with you being unable to go to the toilet even though you may feel you need to.

Therefore, if your bladder or bowel is not functioning as it normally does, it is not necessarily because you are suffering with CES. It may be because of the pain you are in or the medication you are taking. Nevertheless, if you are in any doubt, it is important you seek professional medical advice as soon as possible, starting with your GP or visiting A&E if your GP is not available.

Crumbling Spine

Wow, do I hate this one! More often than not this term is given to people who are suffering with arthritis of the spine (see Arthritis). Therefore, to say it is crumbling is ludicrous and wrong. I have had some patients visit me who have been told this because they are suffering with osteoporosis (see Osteoporosis). Although I can understand why someone with osteoporosis may be told they have a 'crumbling spine', it is once again incorrect to do so. Okay, you may have an increased risk of fractures of the vertebral bodies of the spine, but to say your spine is crumbling is being melodramatic to say the least.

Degeneration

This can be described as referring to deterioration or 'breaking down' and is synonymous with arthritis (see Arthritis).

Degenerative Disc Disease

I can understand how some patients are shaken to the core when they are given the diagnosis of 'Degenerative Disc Disease'. It sounds serious. However, although it can be a cause of pain, it is not as serious as it sounds.

In a nutshell, it is simply wear and tear of the discs, which we will all suffer from as we get older. Therefore, if we are going to be quite literal about it, every one of us is going to develop Degenerative Disc Disease providing we live long enough!

Just because you are suffering with wear and tear of your discs, or any other structure for that matter, it does not necessarily mean it is the cause of your pain or, if it is, that there is nothing we can do to relieve that pain. Please read about arthritis where I explain why I believe having 'wear and tear' does not necessarily mean you need suffer with pain.

Disc Bulge

See Herniated Disc.

Disc Narrowing

This will usually occur as a result of 'Degenerative Disc Disease'. In other words, as the disc is affected by wear and tear, it becomes narrowed. This in turn places more pressure on the facet joints at the back of the vertebra and increases the risk of facet joint pain.

Facet Joint Arthropathy

As mentioned under arthropathy, this is saying there is something wrong with the facet joints, quite often wear and tear.

Fibromyalgia

Website: <http://www.fibromyalgia-associationuk.org>
This is a problem which causes pain in the muscles, ligaments and tendons. However, a great deal is still unknown about this condition, as it is also associated with signs and symptoms such as fatigue, tiredness and headaches.

Due to it affecting the soft tissues mentioned above, all of which are present in the lower back, it can obviously be a cause of low back pain or sciatica. Typically, however, it tends to be quite a widespread pain throughout the body. For further information contact the Fibromyalgia Association UK

Herniated Disc

This is where the middle part of the disc (Nucleus Pulposus) – see the chapter, **Learning Zone: *Your Lower Back and Sciatic Nerve*** – exerts pressure upon the outer layer (Annulus Fibrosus) and therefore creates a 'bulge' or herniation. The disc would typically herniate postero-laterally. If large enough, this can irritate the spinal nerves as they leave the spinal canal and consequently create nerve root pain or 'sciatica', which you may feel down the leg. Although quite rare, a disc can also herniate anteriorly. If it does so, it may compress the Cauda Equina (See Cauda Equina Syndrome)

Idiopathic Back Pain

This could also be termed 'I don't know' back pain. Any diagnosis which uses the term idiopathic is basically saying it is not really known why you are suffering from such a condition.

Lesion

This refers to changes which are 'abnormal', i.e. ideally should not be there. So if you have been diagnosed as having a Disc Lesion, it may be there are some changes taking place in the disc, for example, wear and tear.

Lumbar Spinal Stenosis

This is where the Spinal Canal of the Lumbar Spine becomes narrowed (Stenosis = narrowing). As a result of this narrowing, increased pressure is placed upon the spinal cord. A typical sign of this is increased pain either in the back or down both legs when you are walking, with almost immediate relief if you were to bend forward or sit down, especially in a slumped position. This problem would definitely present as EDP and if you feel this is what you may be suffering with, you need to see your GP.

Although not a medical emergency, it can be very difficult to treat conservatively and therefore the likelihood is you may need an appointment with an orthopaedic consultant.

Muscle Spasm

This is where the muscle contracts involuntary and very harshly. It is more than the muscle simply tightening up, which often occurs with a lot of low back pain.

Nerve Compression

This occurs when abnormal pressure is placed upon a nerve, resulting in it being 'compressed'. This may be a result of, amongst other things, a herniated disc or wear and tear of the facet joints. If this irritation results in inflammation, the patient will experience pain. Nerve compression can also result in pins and needles and/or numbness.

Osteo-Arthritis

See Arthritis.

Osteoporosis

Website: <http://www.nos.org.uk>
This literally means 'porous bones'. Individuals with osteoporosis suffer brittle bones which can be broken more readily than most. However, this does not mean you are going to suffer a fracture, there will be plenty of people walking around suffering with osteoporosis of the spine who will never suffer any kind of fracture, with the condition itself having varying degrees of severity.

People suffering with osteoporosis of the spine often develop a very flexed posture, due to the way the vertebral bodies begin to lose height. They will also appear to lose height themselves.

If you feel you may be suffering with osteoporosis, it is important to visit your GP. You may need a bone scan to determine whether you are osteoporotic. If so, you may need to be prescribed medication and also be given advice with regard to an appropriate exercise programme.

Pinched Nerve

See Nerve Compression.

Prolapsed Disc

See Herniated Disc.

Rheumatoid Arthritis

Website: <http://www.rheumatoid.org.uk>
This is a progressive auto-immune (where the body appears to 'attack' itself) disease. Typically, the hands, feet and wrists are affected and these joints often become hot and swollen; however, it can also affect the spine. The diagnosis is made clinically, i.e. by taking into account your signs and symptoms, along with tests such as from a blood sample.

Sciatica

Another frustration of mine is when a diagnosis is given as 'sciatica'. This is not a diagnostic term, rather a descriptive one. The sciatic nerve passes down the leg – see the chapter, **Learning Zone:** *Your Lower Back and Sciatic Nerve* – and therefore any pain which passes down the leg, which is presumed to come from the lower back or sciatic nerve, is often diagnosed as sciatica. However, the true diagnosis may be a herniated disc or compressed nerve as a result of facet joint arthropathy, two completely different problems that would be treated very differently.

Scoliosis

Website: <http://www.srs.org/patients>
This refers to a sideways curve of the spine. As described in the chapter, **Learning Zone:** *Your Lower Back and Sciatic Nerve*, there is a natural curve in the spine when viewed from the side. However, if you were to look at someone's spine from behind, it should be straight. If it is not straight, however, but rather a curve is present from left to right or vice versa, this is referred to as scoliosis.

I have treated many patients who have been diagnosed with scoliosis, yet it is quite subtle and needs no further intervention apart from an appropriate exercise regime. More often than not, scoliosis can be treated conservatively. If quite severe, however, further intervention may be necessary.

Do not worry yourself unnecessarily though. If you have been diagnosed with scoliosis from an x-ray, there is every chance that:

i) You do not even have scoliosis! Many people with low back pain or sciatica either hold themselves awkwardly due to pain, or any muscle spasm present creates a scoliosis, where the muscles pull tighter on one side of the spine compared to the other. Therefore, under these circumstances, as soon as your pain begins to resolve itself, so too will the scoliosis.

ii) The scoliosis you have is relatively subtle and therefore simple exercises will be enough for it to resolve or for your back to be strong enough to compensate for it.

Therefore, do not worry yourself too much if you feel you have scoliosis. Nevertheless, you should still have it checked by a health professional, so pay your GP a visit.

Slipped Disc

See Disc Herniation.

Spinal Stenosis

See Lumbar Spinal Stenosis.

Spondylolysis

This is where there is a defect in a specific part of the Lumbar vertebra, usually a stress fracture. Spondylolysis is a common cause of Spondylolisthesis.

Spondylolisthesis

This is a condition where one Lumbar vertebra 'slips forward' in relation to an adjacent vertebra. Once again, as I have mentioned with several of the diagnoses given, there may be many people who would present with Spondylolisthesis were they to x-ray their spines, yet they will never know as they will suffer no signs or symptoms.

Those suffering with signs and symptoms as a result of this condition are often treated conservatively with appropriate strengthening exercises. However, if quite severe and the associated signs and symptoms will not resolve, further intervention may be indicated.

Spondylosis

Medical jargon for wear and tear (see Arthritis).

Trapped Nerve

See Nerve Compression.

Wear and Tear

See Arthritis.

Appendix II:

Glossary of Terms

The following is an explanation of any words you may have encountered throughout this book.

Abduction
The movement where any joint/limb (with regard to this book, the hip/leg) is taken away from the body and out to the side. The opposite of Adduction.

Accident and Emergency (A&E)
A&E is the department of a hospital where people are treated with serious injuries and are in need of emergency treatment. They are also known as the Emergency Department (ED), Emergency Room (ER), Emergency Ward (EW) or Casualty in other parts of the world. They are typically open 24 hours a day, 365 days of the year.

Adduction
The movement where any joint/limb (with regard to this book, the hip/leg) is taken back towards the side of body. The opposite of Abduction.

Anterior
The front of your body.

Anterior Rotation
Where the top part of the pelvis moves forwards in relation to the bottom part of the pelvis. For example, if you were in the crook lying position and tried to arch your lower back upwards and away from the floor. The opposite of posterior rotation.

Articular Surface
The surface of each adjacent bone, which make contact with one another to form a joint.

Articulate
To form a joint with, i.e. two bones articulate with each other to form a joint.

Auto-immune
Where the body's own natural immune system does not recognise its own healthy tissue and consequently 'attacks' it.

Bilateral
Applying to both sides, i.e. left and right.

Central/Centrally/Centralising
Moving towards the centre of the body. With reference to sciatica, the pain may travel centrally from the knee towards the lower back. The opposite to distal/distally/peripheralising.

Contra-indications
Where a potential treatment for an ailment is judged to be inadvisable. Usually due to the potential side-effects of that treatment. For example, having an allergy to paracetamol would be a contra-indication to taking paracetamol for your low back pain.

Crook Lying
The position where you lie on your back with your knees bent.

Distal/Distally/Peripheralising
Moving away from the centre of the body. With reference to low back pain and sciatica, the pain may travel distally from the lower back and down the leg. The opposite of Central/Centrally/Centralising.

Extension
With regard to the lower back, this refers to the action of leaning backwards. When in relation to your hip, this is the action of taking your upper leg backwards so as to pass behind you. Extension is the opposite movement to flexion.

Extension Dominated Pain (EDP)

Low back pain or sciatica which is made worse by positions that involve extension of the lower back. The opposite of Flexion Dominated Pain (FDP).

External Rotation/Externally Rotates.

The process of turning a limb out away from the body. With regard to the hip, imagine lying flat on your back and 'rolling' your leg outwards. The opposite of internal rotation/internally rotates.

Flexion

With regard to the lower back, this refers to the action of bending forward, as if to touch your toes. When in relation to your hip, this is the action of bringing your knee up towards your chest. Flexion is the opposite movement to extension.

Flexion Dominated Pain (FDP)

Low back pain or sciatica, which is made worse by positions that involve flexion of the lower back. The opposite of Extension Dominated Pain (EDP).

General Practitioner (GP)

This is the name given to the health professional who is your point of first contact should you become unwell. Also referred to as a Primary Care Physician (PCP) in other parts of the world, or simply your 'Doctor'.

Internal Rotation/Internally Rotates

The process of turning a limb in towards the body. With regard to the hip, imagine lying flat on your back and 'rolling' your leg inwards. The opposite of external rotation/externally rotates.

Kyphosis

The natural curve in the Thoracic Spine when viewed from the side. See the chapter, **Learning Zone:** *Your Lower Back and Sciatic Nerve* for a diagram of the spine.

Kyphotic

Appertaining to Kyphosis.

Lordosis

The natural curve in the Lumbar Spine when viewed from the side. See the chapter, **Learning Zone:** *Your Lower Back and Sciatic Nerve* for a diagram of the spine.

Lordotic

Appertaining to Lordosis.

Musculo-skeletal

Referring to muscles and bones. With regard to this book, low back pain and sciatica primarily caused by problems with muscles and bones.

Nerve Roots

These are where the nerves from the spinal cord leave the vertebral column. The nerve root L1 leaves the vertebral column between the first and second lumbar vertebra, i.e. between L1 and L2. Each nerve root can join other nerve roots to form a peripheral nerve, e.g. the nerve roots of L4–S3 join together to form the sciatic nerve (see the chapter, **Learning Zone:** *Your Lower Back and Sciatic Nerve* for a diagram of the spinal cord and associated nerve roots.)

Orthotics

With reference to the foot, an insole placed inside the shoe to correct any mal-alignment that may be present.

Paraesthesia

Abnormal skin sensation.

Peripheralising

See Distal/Distally/Peripheralising.

Placebo

Where a treatment is administered that is not believed to have any direct effect on the patient's condition.

Podiatrist

A person medically trained to treat disorders of the foot/lower limb.

Posterior

The back of your body.

Posterior Rotation

Where the top part of the pelvis moves backwards in relation to the bottom part of the pelvis. For example, if you were in the crook lying position and tried to flatten your lower back into the floor. The opposite of anterior rotation.

Postero-lateral

To move backwards and also to the side. The typical position a prolapsed disc tends to take – see the chapter, **Learning Zone: *Your Lower Back and Sciatic Nerve***.

Prone Lying

Lying on your stomach.

Rotation

Twisting/turning to one side.

Side flexion

Side bending your body to one side, as if sliding your arm down the side of your leg.

Soft tissue

The structures including, but not exclusive to, muscles, ligaments and nerves.

Supine Lying

Lying on your back.

Unilateral

Applying to one side only, i.e. the left or right.